The Antibiotic Paradox

THE ANTIBIOTIC PARADOX

How the Misuse of Antibiotics Destroys Their Curative Powers

STUART B. LEVY, M.D.

PERSEUS
PUBLISHING

Many of the designations used by manufacturers and sellers to distinguish their products are claimed as trademarks. Where those designations appear in this book and Perseus Publishing was aware of a trademark claim, the designations have been printed in initial capital letters.

Copyright © 2002 by Stuart B. Levy, M.D.

Cataloging-in-Publication Data is available from the Library of Congress
ISBN 0-7382-0440-4

Perseus Publishing is a member of the Perseus Books Group.

Find us on the World Wide Web at http://www.perseuspublishing.com

Perseus Publishing books are available at special discounts for bulk purchases in the U.S. by corporations, institutions, and other organizations. For more information, please contact the Special Markets Department at the Perseus Books Group, 11 Cambridge Center, Cambridge, MA 02142, or call (800) 255-1514 or (617) 252-5298, or e-mail j.mccrary@perseusbooks.com.

Set in 11-point Janson by Perseus Publishing Services

First printing, December 2001

EBC   02 03 04 05   13 12 11 10 9 8 7 6 5 4 3

*To Suzanne, Arthur, and Walter
and all future generations*

Preface to
the Second Edition

Since the publication of this book in 1992, there have been a number of encouraging developments aimed at resolving the antibiotic resistance problem. There is greater public awareness of antibiotic resistance and the need for new antibiotics. Many large pharmaceutical companies have re-entered the field, either by reconstituting their infectious disease units or by establishing ties with smaller biotechnology companies whose work shows promise toward finding novel antibiotics. Government and nongovernment health organizations have found alliances to confront the mounting public health crisis.

On the negative side, the situation *vis a vis* resistance has not diminished, but has continued to increase, with the appearance of vancomycin-resistant forms of methicillin-resistant staphylococci and the emergence of increasing numbers of bacterial strains resistant to all, or almost all, the currently available antibiotics. Of recent concern, consumers have sought out antibacterial-containing cleaning products for their homes, raising the specter of yet other means of selecting resistant strains and altering the kinds of microbes found in homes and around us.

As antibiotic resistance continued to increase, no new antibiotic was approved, until late 1999–early 2000. Two new ones were released for hospital-acquired gram-positive infections, namely staphylococci and enterococci. These drugs serve a long-awaited need in the cure of some otherwise untreatable infections. But other ominous bacteria with resistance to all antibiotics still loom on the horizon and no other new antibiotics are expected soon. While we have begun the 21st century with increased activity in the anti-infective field, we are still faced with immediate need for new drugs and more prudent management of antibiotics to curb resistance in our communities and health care institutions.

The year 2001 was a watershed year for establishing public health initiatives to address antibiotic resistance. The World Health Organization cited antibiotic resistance as one of the three major public health threats of the next 21st century and developed a global action plan to contain antibiotic resistance. The WHO general assembly of 125 nations pledged efforts to curtail the problem in countries worldwide. Major national and international societies have issued statements and established special programs to confront antibiotic resistance. The American College of Physicians–American Society of Internal Medicine and the American Academy of Pediatrics published guidelines for physicians, urging more rational prescription of antibiotics to preserve their efficacy. The *Alliance for the Prudent Use of Antibiotics* (APUA), celebrating its 20th anniversary in 2001, released a 350-page report that summarized and reviewed 25 documents from worldwide experts in the area of antibiotic resistance over the past 15 years. Commissioned by the World Health Organization, it supports the WHO's *Global Strategy on Containment of Antimicrobial Resistance* by defining the factors leading to antibiotic resistance and the approaches recommended by the expert groups. Both documents stress the worldwide nature of the problem and the need for both local and global action.

The veterinary medical community and human medical teams are starting to talk about achieving understanding of the mutual need for antibiotics and the negative consequences that both animal and human misuse have on the pool of resistant bacteria. The U.S. Food and Drug Administration has put together a Framework Document as a basis for discussion and implementation of guidelines for the approval of new antibiotics and their use in animals. While antibiotic use is certainly the pervading, major factor in the emergence of resistance, resistant strains persist even after antibiotics have been withdrawn. This recognition defines the "post-antibiotic" survival of these resistant bacteria, which then take on a "life of their own." Therefore, we need to prevent the emergence of resistance in the first place through more prudent use of existing agents. Once "let out of the barn," resistance is hard to contain.

While the focus of antibiotic testing has been directed at clinical isolates, studies now begin to examine harmless so-called "commensal bacteria" for the presence of antibiotic resistance. These organisms constitute the larger reservoir of resistance genes. Their frequency of resistance serves both as a barometer of antibiotic use and a measure of its consequences, as well as an indication of sources of antibiotic resistance genes for pathogens of animals, people, and plants. An APUA website and list-serv called ROAR currently provides a forum for comments on the concept of "reservoirs of antibiotic resistance."

As we begin the new century, the unfolding picture is one of ubiquitous resistance genes. There is a need to track these resistance genes and bacteria in order to guide clinical practice, serve as an early warning of emerging resistance, and help analyze patterns to inform drug developments and innovations. International systems for surveillance of resistance among the clinical isolates emerged in the previous decade. Two are sponsored by drug companies (SENTRY from Bristol Myers Squibb and Alexander Project from GlaxoSmithKline) and another, TSN, from Focus Technologies. These constitute the first formal efforts at determining the worldwide frequency of antibiotic resistance according to the type of bacteria and antibiotic. Interestingly, while cynics argue that there has been an exaggeration of the frequency of resistance, the surveillance systems have revealed an even greater resistance problem than previously surmised. APUA has established a collaborative effort among these three groups and other surveillance systems under GAARD (Global Alliance of Antibiotic Resistance Data), which, in addition to its advisory role, collects and disseminates data on resistance frequencies.

In an unprecedented move, ten agencies of the U.S. government joined together to put forth an Interagency Plan to combat antibiotic resistance. In a comprehensive program with over 80 action items, each agency has adopted segments of the problem to address. The U.S. government has issued a legislative initiative to increase funds to augment the public health infrastructures that confront the antibiotic resistance problem. While these directives fortify current efforts to curtail antibiotic resistance, it is clear that much more needs to be done.

There is also a greater appreciation that antibiotics need to be used in an environmentally "neutral" fashion, i.e., to maintain susceptible flora as natural competitors against invading resistant strains. Resistance is a natural consequence of antibiotic use, but the *persistence* of resistant strains in an environment is dependent on their ability to out-compete the native susceptible flora.

Antibiotics are unique therapeutics. Any individual use affects the microbial environment and thereby society. Emergence of antibiotic resistance is a subsequent problem not only for the individual, but also for others sharing the environment. For this reason, I propose that antibiotics be given their own drug category through regulatory agencies. Such an action will put emphasis on the consequences that individual misuse of antibiotics has on society at large. Such categorization will allow special considerations for these drugs in terms of how they are used, how they are marketed, and how their efficacy can be preserved through incentives provided to industry and education given to producers and consumers.

Given the tragic events of September 11, 2001, antibiotics take on even further critical importance as treatment and prophylaxis of diseases stemming from a bioterrorist attack. Since resistance determinants to all currently available antibiotics are known, even a basic geneticist could engineer a variety of these genes into disease agents. Therefore, it becomes exceedingly crucial to understand the mechanisms for resistance and how to overcome them. We need to know what quantities of which antibiotics (and vaccines) which will effectively neutralize the deployed biological weapons that are currently available. In this regard, new antibiotics are sorely needed to further assure our ability to curtail such an attack.

In sum, much has happened in the nearly 10 years since the first publication of this book. Antibiotics still wreak havoc by selecting resistant organisms, but we know more about the problem and the factors that drive it. The paradox remains. In a perverse way, antibiotics select for the kinds of bacteria that they can no longer kill. But recognition of the problem and commitment to control it are growing among influential groups worldwide. There is a much broader consensus of the need to intervene and alter the current course. There is even brighter optimism for the future as pharmaceutical companies renew efforts to discover new drugs and individuals begin concerted efforts to control and reverse this public health problem.

Prudent use of antibiotics requires an understanding of and foresight into the environmental consequences of antibiotic use. Susceptible bacteria are important allies in controlling the invasion and propagation of resistant bacteria. The aim of the current and future use of antibiotics should be the revival and maintenance of the normal susceptible microbial flora.

Stuart B. Levy, M.D.
Boston, Massachusetts

Preface to
the First Edition

Antibiotics have been called the single most important therapeutic discovery in the history of medicine. While other medications could compete for this distinction, antibiotics as a
class have clearly revolutionized our ability to curb death and
disease from infectious microorganisms. An interesting feature of their historic discoveries is that they occurred within
the lifetime of many of the population living today.

The ability of antibiotics, such as penicillin, to effect rapid
cures for previously fatal infections led to their being touted
as "miracle drugs." This claim remains today, having been
passed down through several recent generations. While, to
some extent, antibiotics have merited this appellation, it paradoxically has caused some dent in their armor. The seemingly
endless miracles attributed to these drugs have led to their
misuse and overuse. Bacteria responded to the widespread application of antibiotics by finding ways to become resistant, in
other words, insensitive to the killing effects of these powerful
drugs.

Thus, antibiotics sow the seeds of their own potential
downfall by selecting for rare strains of bacteria that have the
ability to resist their activity. To complicate matters further,
many of these resistance traits can be transferred or spread

from one kind of resistant bacteria to other bacteria, even of different types.

This adverse result of antibiotic use, a phenomenon that I call the "antibiotic paradox," does not mean that antibiotics have failed or that antibiotics cannot still be used. It simply reflects the dual nature of the powerful effects they have and why they should be used prudently. Fortunately, antibiotics remain very effective in the treatment of a vast majority of bacterial infectious diseases. This situation, however, is not secure and is changing continually. In many parts of the world, cost-effective, inexpensive, and safe antibiotics are no longer successful because of the bacterial resistance to them that has developed. Effective treatment is absent in many parts of the world where newer drugs developed to treat resistant bacteria are too expensive to be made available on the limited national budgets of these developing countries. Therefore, the older antibiotics continue to be used despite growing resistance patterns and, in turn, continue to propagate new and often more resistant types of bacteria. Also, the distribution of these drugs is often uneven. In some areas, antibiotics are being overused, while in other areas, often those needing them the most, they are drastically underused because of a lack of availability. Hence, the general "use" of antibiotics needs improvement in all parts of the world.

The aim of this book is to explain where and when antibiotics are useful and why they are so valuable. On the other side, there are various uses of antibiotics that should be changed and even curtailed. Our goal is not to suggest the removal of antibiotics from the physician's armamentarium but, in fact, to encourage making them even *more* effective by curbing the emergence and spread of resistant forms of infectious bacteria.

This goal of improving antibiotic use must concern all members of society using these drugs, namely: consumers, whether they be humans, animals, or the agriculture industry; prescribers, whether they be physicians, veterinarians, or plant pathologists; and the producers and companies that are making and marketing these drugs. By recognizing the different areas in which antibiotic use can be improved, we can hope to stimulate better distribution and application, increase awareness of the benefits to be reaped, and curb the threat posed by resistance. The worldwide aim is to protect the effectiveness of these precious natural resources.

Stuart B. Levy, M.D.
Boston, Massachusetts

Acknowledgments

I thank Linda Regan, Victoria Cherney, and Naomi Brier of Plenum Publishing Corporation for their important insights, suggestions, and probing questions, which helped me put these thoughts together and kept me on the path, aware of my audience. Much appreciated were their continued interest and encouragement.

I am particularly grateful to my long-term associate Bonnie Marshall for her immense help during the final stages of this project, including repeated editing of the test and the superb rendition of the concepts into pictures and graphics. I thank Herbert Hächler, another one of those rare scientists with an artist's flair, for his "made-to-order" cartoons that are on target and certainly liven up the text.

I greatly appreciate the help and information received from Anne Vidaver, Thomas Sullivan, Margaret Erwin, Hachiro Shimanuchi, Howard Myers, Charles Bramble, and Neil Pelletier, in the preparation of the sections dealing with non-human uses of antibiotics. I thank Cameron Macauley for his help in researching the material for Chapter 1 and Peter Steere for assistance in the pharmaceutical details.

I also thank those who contributed photographs, in particular Angelo dePaola, who also shared the catfish operation with me as well as so many of the interesting details about raising catfish.

I appreciate the hospitality of Mr. Richard Wolfe of the rare
books section of the Countway Medical Library, where I was
able to gather so much first-hand material dealing with the
history of medicine.

Special thanks go to Claire Sherman, Anne Ryan, Kenneth
Ratzan, Jay Levy, Stephen Beal, and Patricia Suzman for their
helpful comments on the text.

I particularly thank my wife, Cecile, for her loving support
throughout this venture, and my laboratory for providing
me with the interesting experimental results relating to this
subject.

In the preparation of the second edition of this book, I deeply
thank Bonnie Marshall for her invaluable and continued assistance in both the editing of the text and the production of new
figures. Once again I thank Herbert Hächler for answering my
call to convert scientific concepts into exceptional cartoons. I
thank Andrew Prazar, my assistant, for his tireless efforts in
putting this material into shape through seemingly endless revisions, Eduardo Robleto and Teresa Barbosa for help in the
design of figures, and the staff at Perseus Books for their pa-
tience in handling my revisions. I appreciate the help from
Gerald Johnson of the University of Prince Edward Island, Se-
bastian Bell from the Maine Aquaculture Center, Robert Bayer
of the University of Maine, and Thomas Bell of the United
States Fish and Wildlife Service in providing updated information about antibiotic use in aquaculture (Chapter 7). I thank the
research scientists working with me over the past thirty years at
Tufts University School of Medicine for their dedicated efforts
towards helping us understand the genetics, biochemistry, and
ecology of antibiotic resistance. Their discoveries and insights
form an important basis for the messages and ideas presented
in this book. Thanks to my wife Cecile and my children
Suzanne, Arthur, and Walter for supporting me with love and
understanding in preparing this new edition.

Contents

chapter one

From Tragedy the Antibiotic Age is Born

"450 DIE AS FLAMES AND PANIC TRAP COCOANUT GROVE CROWD . . . "[1] screamed the headlines of the *Boston Herald* on Sunday morning, November 29, 1942, filling almost the entire top half of the front page (Figure 1.1, next page). The *Boston Sunday Globe* likewise flashed "400 DEAD IN HUB NIGHTCLUB FIRE. HUNDREDS HURT IN PANIC AS THE COCOANUT GROVE BECOMES WILD INFERNO."[2] This was the most devastating fire in the history of Boston and the worst in America since Chicago's Iroquois Theater disaster in 1903, which killed 575 people. The Cocoanut Grove disaster could have been even worse had not advances in medical treatment in the previous 40 years helped in the survival of many victims.

The fire also occasioned a medical event now regarded as historically momentous as the fire itself—the trial of a new, unique drug available only through government sources. Limited amounts of "penicillin," an unknown substance, were released to quell many of the infections contracted by sur-

Figure 1.1. *"The fire that made penicillin famous." It was in treating victims of this Boston fire that penicillin had its first large and publicized clinical trial. The mystery surrounding this "priceless substance" and its acclaimed remarkable powers pushed the United States government and American companies to proceed with its mass production* (The Boston Herald).

vivors of the fire. Until then, the public had little or no conception of this drug's success in treating and preventing life-threatening infections.

The Cocoanut Grove was one of a number of entertainment establishments in Boston, like many in other cities throughout the country, where people went to get away from the agonies and disappointments of World War II that confronted them daily. Over its 15-year history, the club had maintained its reputation as "the" place to be and to be seen. That Saturday night had been no exception.

The club was teeming with its biggest crowd ever. An estimated 800 to 1,000 people crammed its rooms. Servicemen in town for a weekend of relaxation conversed with the locals. Fans from Holy Cross College were there to celebrate after an upset football victory over Boston College. By a certain irony, the Boston College team players were spared the tragedy. Discouraged by their loss, they had gone to bed early, foregoing the evening's planned festivities at the Cocoanut Grove.

The nightclub was located at Piedmont Street and Shawmut Avenue in Boston's South End, adjoining the theater district. Crucial to the chaos that immediately followed the first sign of fire was the single revolving door entrance on Piedmont Street, which led into the main foyer. It was here that hundreds of customers scrambled to get out, only to be crushed and then suffocated in the panic. The nightclub's tenor, Billy Payne, saved ten customers by leading them into the basement icebox and later out to safety. He had been scheduled to open the show with the "Star Spangled Banner" when a screaming young woman who was afire stopped the show. Some found refuge on the roof, but most people were trapped inside.

The crowd was in full regalia at the time the fire started, a tragic accident ignited by a young barboy with a lighted match. In an interview that night he told a *Boston Globe* reporter, "I was standing in the dining room talking to the bartender. . . . everything seemed to be all right. . . . all of a sudden, a palm tree, one of those phony ones, went up in flames right before our eyes. I never saw anything like it."[3] By the next day this 16-year-old found out that he was the linchpin of the tragedy.

For days, news of the fire filled the front pages of both city newspapers, relegating even the war to secondary status. More prominent were long lists of those injured in the fire, as well as tallies of the dead and headlines like "Where Bodies Can Be Found."

The majority of the more than 400 victims were taken to the two large city hospitals, while the others were distributed among ten smaller ones for treatment. The havoc at these hospitals necessitated sorting the victims, initially into living and dead and then into those needing limited or more extensive treatment. More than half the victims who arrived were dead or died within five minutes of their arrival. Of the 114 people arriving at the Massachusetts General Hospital, 75 were dead. In all the hospitals, an estimated 200 went directly to the morgue.

Physicians caring for the more than 200 victims who survived the first 24 hours saved more lives than recorded previously for fire victims. They attributed this success to two recent medical therapies. One was an antibacterial, sulfadiazine, a member of the then relatively new class of infectious-disease-killing agents, the sulfonamides, which controlled potentially lethal blood infections caused by the bacterium *Streptococcus*. The other was blood plasma, which was given intravenously to these victims to counteract dehydration caused by fluid loss from the burned surfaces.

Plasma is the fluid part of blood in which the red and white blood cells of the body circulate. Plasma helps maintain a healthy water content in the tissues of the body. The skin is a major protective organ that also maintains balanced body water and temperature. Small amounts of water lost through evaporation through the skin are made up by daily intake of fluids. When the skin is destroyed, as in a severe burn, large losses of water and plasma occur, which can lead to shock and death. In this instance, fluid replacement by mouth is not rapid enough nor sufficient to prevent the potentially fatal consequences.

Almost three-quarters of the burn victims who survived the initial 24 hours sustained large fluid losses through their burns. By giving back plasma, doctors were able to replace lost fluid and body salts, avoiding severe dehydration, shock, and death for an estimated 150 burn victims. At the time of the fire, the technology for separating plasma from blood cells and supplying it for injection into the bloodstream was only four years old. Thus, Cocoanut Grove burn victims were among the first to benefit from this new therapy. A total of 1,300 units, taken from 1,300 donors, were used during this critical period in the treatment of burn victims.

Yet another new medical treatment, virtually unknown at the time, appeared at one hospital. The Massachusetts General Hospital received a new drug that was made available for use in preventing fatal infections by other bacteria. According to the December 2, 1942, issue of *The Boston Globe*, Merck and Company in Rahway, New Jersey, rushed a 32-liter supply of a "priceless" drug to the Massachusetts General Hospital. With police escorts, it made a 7-hour, 368-mile drive through four states in steady rain from its New Jersey production site to the hospital.[4] The drug was penicillin, not in pure form, but actually delivered in the culture liquid in which the drug was produced by a *Penicillium* mold. It combatted *Staphylococcus aureus*, a frequent bacterial contaminant of skin wounds of fire victims.

Once the protective skin is damaged, staphylococci can enter the body, where they circulate and multiply in the bloodstream, leading to high fevers, shock, and death. Prior to the Cocoanut Grove fire, there were no agents readily available to treat this bacterium. Once infections occurred, most patients died. Staphylococci were also the cause of failure of skin grafts, since the microorganisms set up infections on the exposed skin surfaces. The trial use of this new drug presaged its future significance.

Penicillin was described officially as a "medical safeguard against infection." It was still a highly guarded secret and was reserved for military use only. But for victims of this fire, it was released by the government in what became one of its most important clinical trials. The success of skin grafting and treating the severely burned patients was largely attributed to the action of penicillin. This single event has been labeled "crucial" in prompting the United States government to back pharmaceutical houses in their production of penicillin in large amounts.

The enticement of the United States into pursuing penicillin—which has been called a British discovery—followed diplomacy and persistence by the drug's leading developer and protagonist, Howard Florey. Although he did not discover penicillin—that honor goes to a fellow countryman, Alexander Fleming—he and his colleagues are credited with producing it and with demonstrating the drug's success in therapy. Florey, along with Norman Heatley, his colleague and fellow chemist, had made a special trip from England to the United States in the summer of 1941 to expound the wonders of penicillin and to persuade the United States government to back large-scale production. Florey and his team saw this effort as essential for treating casualties of the war abroad and at home, but the financial constraints caused by the war made production impossible for Great Britain. The Cocoanut Grove fire occurred about a year after the visit by these British scientists. Although small amounts of penicillin had been made available and were used successfully in a limited number of patients in the United States, no United States commitment toward production of the drug had been made. During the year since the British visit, other American physicians had received small amounts of the precious new substance and reported "miraculous" results. The glowing reports made the large pharmaceutical houses aware of the new compound's powers. Still, there was hesitation in putting the huge amount of resources needed behind production of a relatively unknown entity. Moreover, giving people penicillin, a natural product of a microorganism, still seemed a questionable idea.

Penicillin's use in treating some of the victims of the Cocoanut Grove tragedy received far more attention than the number of patients treated. Still, very little penicillin was available. Fewer than 100 people in the United States had been treated with it before the fire. It was difficult to purify and its full effects were not known. Drug manufacturers and the United States government demanded proof of its worth and lack of toxicity before mass production could be initiated. The national attention brought to penicillin by the "infamous disaster" did the job. Certainly it was thanks to other medical measures that so many victims lived. But the media focused special attention on the new drug, penicillin. The news accounts provided a widely publicized forum for relating its unknown prior successes, namely, accounts of treated patients who were cured of life-threatening infections. Meanwhile, the enthusiasm for producing penicillin reached new heights.

Penicillin earned the accolade "miracle drug" because of its unique and rapid control of infectious bacteria that, before penicillin's discovery, had been fully expected to kill the patient. Small amounts of the drug cured blood-borne infections, pneumonias, and open skin wounds. The discovery of sulfonamides in the mid-1930s had revived the quest for what the 19th-century German chemist Paul Ehrlich called a "magic bullet," that is, a drug that would kill bacterial invaders without harming the body. Penicillin seemed to be the epitome of the concept. It killed bacteria that the sulfonamides could not affect and produced fewer side effects. It maintained its activity while penetrating dying tissue, a feature that no other drug had demonstrated. Penicillin clearly symbolized our ability to outwit and control the microbial world. Ironically, the drug itself was not man-made, but a product of molds—natural participants of the microbial environment. For such naturally occurring substances that killed bacteria, the term "antibiotic" was coined.

Amidst the deserved optimism surrounding the successes of penicillin, hovered words of caution. The British bacteriologist Alexander Fleming, who discovered the drug, warned in a 1945 interview by the *New York Times* that misuse of penicillin could lead to the selection and propagation of mutant forms of bacteria resistant to the drug. He had derived such mutant bacteria in the laboratory by growing susceptible bacterial

strains in increasingly higher amounts of penicillin, starting
with very small amounts of the drug. These mutant bacteria
had cell walls that were much less permeable to penicillin, so
the drug could not penetrate the bacteria and kill them.
These bacteria could resist the levels of penicillin that normally circulated in the blood during treatment with the drug.
Fleming, hoping to avoid producing these mutants in patients
during therapy, spoke out for complete courses of treatment,
since inadequate treatments were more likely to select for,
and lead to overgrowth of, these resistant forms.

Fleming predicted that this situation would be worse when
the drug became available in an oral form. Then it could be
taken easily by patients in their homes without the necessity
of intravenous therapy, which required hospitalization. Drug
use was monitored in hospitals. On the outside, this would be
hard to do. He warned the medical world that

> the greatest possibility of evil in self-medication is the use of
> too small doses so that instead of clearing up infection, the mi-
> crobes are educated to resist penicillin and a host of penicillin-
> fast organisms is bred out which can be passed to other individ-
> uals and from them to others until they reach someone who
> gets a septicemia or a pneumonia which penicillin cannot save.[5]

These early words predicted a phenomenon, namely, that
resistant bacteria would be selected by misuse of antibiotics
and that resistant strains selected in one person, who might
remain unaffected, could spread to another. The other person
could come down with a form of the disease now insensitive
to penicillin. Nevertheless, there was great interest in providing medications that could be given by mouth. Intravenous
therapy was not as convenient then as it is today. Hospitals
did not have the sterile plastic tubings and disposable needles
we have now. Intravenous therapy required reusable materials

that had to be sterilized after every use. The availability of oral medications would avoid these cumbersome necessities and make treatments far easier.

When the drug became available orally, it was a major breakthrough, but as Fleming warned, it was also a sure invitation for misuse. Until the mid-1950s, it was available without a doctor's advice. The drug appeared in over-the-counter preparations and was advertised to the public (Figure 1.2, next page). This free access to penicillin led to its use for diseases not responsive to antibiotics. Moreover, even if there were a bacterial cause, a patient taking less than an optimal dosage would not totally eradicate the infectious agent. Bacteria surviving the incomplete treatment could continue to multiply and among them would be mutants with less susceptibility to the antibiotic—like the ones Fleming produced in the laboratory.

But Alexander Fleming's predictions were borne out in a more devastating way than even he surmised. He did not imagine, nor did anyone else at the time, that mutations were not the only way by which bacteria could become resistant. Rare traits already existed in nature that enabled the bacteria not only to resist the drug but to actually destroy it. Proteins for destroying penicillin made bacteria much more resistant to penicillin than did the cell wall mutants that Fleming produced in the laboratory. The synthesis of these proteins was dictated by genetic material, that is, genes, newly acquired by these bacteria. Penicillin resistance genes, harbored in small numbers of bacteria, were soon found in others, meaning that they could be transferred among the bacteria. As a result, each new progeny becomes a resistant one and a potential donor of resistance traits to new recipient bacteria. Under optimal growth conditions, one resistant bacterium can reproduce itself in less than an hour. Thus, in a matter of hours, thousands

Figure 1.2. *When penicillin was first introduced it was not a prescription drug. It was not until the mid-1950s that prescriptions were required. Many companies advertised penicillin to the general public as soon as enough became available. This advertisement appeared in the August 14, 1944, issue of* Life *magazine.*

of copies of the original bacterium, and those that received the resistance gene, can emerge.

The rapid appearance of penicillin-resistant staphylococci sobered the euphoria that followed the discovery of penicillin. In London, these penicillin-destroying staphylococci appeared in hospitals where much of the early use of penicillin had taken place. By one account in 1946, just a few years after the introduction of penicillin, 14% of the strains isolated from sick patients were resistant. By the end of that decade, the frequency had jumped to 59% in the same hospital. Initially, and for the ensuing decade, these resistant strains were concentrated in city hospitals. Then, through the 1960s and 1970s they began to surface elsewhere—first in community hospitals and then among strains from people living in those communities.

The success of penicillin encouraged scientists to search for and discover new antibiotics that could treat other bacteria, including penicillin-resistant strains. Chemists developed the means to modify penicillin so that it was not subject to the enzymes that degraded penicillin. As more antibiotics were discovered, from the late 1940s into the 1970s, the problem of resistance seemed little more than an annoyance. Most major human disease agents remained susceptible to many of the common antibiotics or to other new ones. Then, two events in the mid-1970s marked a dramatic change in this complacent mindset. Two different kinds of common infectious bacteria, one that causes ear infections and meningitis in children and another that causes the venereal disease gonorrhea, emerged with resistance to penicillin. These events occurred in patients in two different parts of the world.

Two infants, 12 and 18 months old, were hospitalized with meningitis in the Naval Hospital in Bethesda, Maryland, one in late 1973 and the other in early 1974. The suspect organism was *Hemophilus influenzae* and the infants were given ampicillin, a penicillin derivative. They died two days later. No one would have expected resistance to this antibiotic since *Hemophilus* bacteria were known to be exceptionally susceptible to ampicillin. In these two patients, however, the *Hemophilus* strains did not respond to the drug. The children, who went to the same day-care center, had picked up strains that were highly resistant, an event that was unexpected after decades of successful ampicillin use. These unique strains had acquired the ability to destroy ampicillin and other related penicillins.

The long-waged war against the ancient scourge, gonorrhea, was presumably over when the early trials with penicillin in the 1940s showed that just a single injection of a small amount of the drug could effectively kill the microorganism. Penicillin could also cure syphilis, another venereal disease often occurring in the same individual. Thus, a single drug could treat two infectious agents potentially present in the same person. But in the mid-1970s, 30 years of success came to a halt. About the same time as *Hemophilus influenzae* appeared with penicillin resistance, so did *Neisseria gonorrhoeae*, the bacteria causing gonorrhea. The resistant strains were also able to destroy the drug. In fact, the enzyme in *N. gonorrhoeae* that destroyed penicillin was the same one found in *H. influenzae*. The identical gene had been picked up by these two different kinds of bacteria. The resistant gonococci were initially discovered in ill servicemen in the Philippines and traced to brothels in Vietnam where penicillin had been given on a regular basis to keep the women "free of disease." Scientists believe that this constant flow of penicillin led to the emergence of rare, never-before-encountered, resistant forms. Since the strains were not contained early enough, they travelled, presumably with infected individuals and with nonsymptomatic human carriers of the bacteria, to the United States and Europe. Today penicillin-resistant gonorrhea strains plague every country of the world.

Figure 1.3.   *The discovery of penicillin led to considerable confidence in winning the fight against bacteria. This dream was short-lived with the emergence of bacterial strains resistant to the drug, first in hospitals and then in the community. While the first round was won by human ingenuity, round two looked like a win for bacteria (Herbert Hächler, University of Zurich, Zurich, Switzerland).*

We can no longer expect that any infection will be cured by the first antibiotic chosen. In some parts of the world, limited supplies of antibiotics mean that *no* available antibiotic is effective. This is a far cry from the situation just 20 years ago. Resistance takes its toll in deaths where newer antibiotics are unavailable or in patients in whom an antibiotic's side effects preclude its use. Patients are suffering and dying from diseases that some predicted 50 years ago would be wiped off the face of the earth. Clearly, the battle we wage with microbes, initially considered won by our enlarging pharmacy of antibiotics, was not an all-out victory for either side (Figure 1.3).

What is the relationship between the use of antibiotics and the emergence of these resistant forms of bacteria? How do these resistance traits find their bacterial hosts and vice versa? How do we, the consumer or the physician, participate in what appears to be a seesaw experience with bacteria—first a win and then a loss? No matter what we do, the bacteria seem to be able to fight back. These are critical questions at a time when bacteria worldwide are becoming resistant to many different antimicrobial agents. Some strains are resistant to all available drugs. To make matters worse, there are no truly new families of antibiotics that we can expect in the immediate future. This means we must make better use of the antibiotics that we already have.

chapter two

The Disease and the Cure

The Microscopic World of Bacteria and Antibiotics

As we go about our everyday activities, we are continually interacting with free-living, single-cell microorganisms invisible to the naked eye. In 1674, a Dutch dry goods merchant, Anton van Leeuwenhoeck, first viewed tiny creatures, "wee animalcules," moving under his hand-sized, homemade microscope. He reported and described his novel findings in letters and drawings, which he sent in 1676 to the Royal Society of London. His discovery opened our eyes and our minds to the existence of living matter that could not normally be seen by the eye. These microscopic beings made up an exotic, previously unimagined world that shared our environment.

But it would take 200 more years before the scientific world would accept bacteria as anything more than interesting creations of nature. That microorganisms could cause illness, the basis of the "germ theory of disease," remained a controversial idea well into the middle of the 19th century. By then, support of the concept was mounting, largely through the ob-

servations and tenacious arguments of Louis Pasteur, who was
working in Paris. He reported that these bacteria, "microbes,"
as the French physician Charles Sedillot suggested in 1878,
were not spontaneously generated from matter, but were present in the air and from there settled onto exposed living tissue, causing it to decompose. His work and theory were accepted and endorsed formally in a statement by the French
Academy of Sciences in 1864. Through his findings and carefully prepared experiments, the French chemist set infectious
disease on a totally new path and ultimately completely altered our views of disease. This major revelation occurred a
little over 100 years ago.

With Pasteur's discoveries and interpretations, scientists
could begin to understand other events in the environment in
a new way. Not only the mystery surrounding the decay of
living tissue but the role of microbes in food production became clear. It was the activity of microscopic beings that
caused juices to turn to wine and bread to rise. This understanding paved the way for new breakthroughs in the food industry. More importantly, this discovery of bacteria as active
participants in mankind's environment allowed them to be
considered as causative agents of human disease.

As the germ theory of disease gained acceptance, scientists
discovered that infectious agents were the cause of many well-
known illnesses whose treatment had been directed previously at multiple symptoms and organs. There evolved a new
recognition that a single microorganism could cause an affliction of many organs of the body. The same disease-causing
agent could bring about chills, fever, and also sore throat. For
the first time, physicians could link a patient's complaints, formerly described in terms of pains and discomforts, to a microbial cause. Diarrhea was caused by certain toxin-forming bacteria that entered the intestinal tract. Burning on urination
occurred because of the irritation of the bladder and urethra
created by bacteria growing there. Bacteria could be found

and identified in the urine. Cough and difficulty in breathing, along with fever and malaise, could be attributed to a single bacterial cause whose most important effect was on the lung, leading to the disease known as pneumonia.

In 1881, Robert Koch furthered diagnostic and medical knowledge by introducing a solid medium in plates on which to grow and distinguish bacteria. This inventive country physician devised this potato extract, a gelatin and agar mixture, in his home kitchen in Germany. He surmised, and later showed, that a single bacterium would stick to a site on the hardened agar surface where it would multiply to form a colony of hundreds of millions of progeny after overnight incubation (Figure 2.1, next page). Each colony on the artificial medium represented the progeny from a single viable microbe. Bacterial types could be determined in urine, feces, sputum, and other clinical specimens taken from the patient. By diluting and plating specimens on the agar surface and counting the colonies after overnight incubation, he could determine the number of microorganisms present.

Scientists distinguished these colonies by their shapes, texture (smooth or rough borders), size, and color (such as translucent, white, red, or yellow). The progeny of the same type of bacteria formed the same kind of colony, but different bacteria formed different colonies. With this method, the medical world finally had a truly objective way to distinguish among various bacterial types. In this way, physicians could begin to identify bacteria and associate a specific bacterial type with a particular disease. Koch's contributions to this budding field did not stop there. He went on to show that a single type of bacterium, isolated and reinoculated into animals, produced the same disease that afflicted animals from which it had come. He is credited with identifying and proving that cholera was caused by a comma-shaped bacterium he had discovered and that tuberculosis was caused by the tubercle bacillus, which he also isolated. This was solid proof of the

Figure 2.1. *This is a modern-day version of the gelatin/agar plate originally developed by Robert Koch in 1881. It is used for the isolation and enumeration of bacteria. Each visible colony, a dot on the plate, represents hundreds of millions of progeny of a single bacterium that landed on the plate prior to overnight incubation.*

role of these bacteria in these diseases and that one bacterial type alone could produce a myriad of signs and symptoms involving multiple organs. The recognition that bacteria cause varied symptoms in *acute* diseases is mirrored by the more recent identification of bacteria as causes of *chronic* diseases, such as the involvement of *Helicobacter pylori* in ulcers.

Bacteria and the Diverse Microbial World

Bacteria are independently multiplying microscopic single-cell organisms. We can safely state that, unlike angels, thousands can sit on the head of a pin. While we can observe them under a 1,000-fold magnification of the microscope (Figure 2.2), even at this enlargement they resemble specks, the size of small dust particles that we see dancing in front of headlights or around illuminated light bulbs. Under much higher magnification, such as with an electron microscope, they appear much more clearly. One million bacteria are still invisible in a milliliter of liquid. Only when 10–100 million bacteria are present does the liquid become turbid.

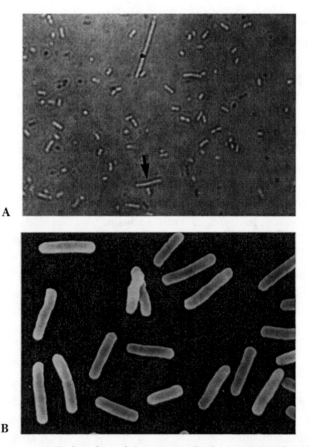

A

B

Figure 2.2. A) Escherichia coli *bacteria visualized at approximately 1000-fold magnification under the phase microscope. Arrow points to one bacterium seen from its side. They appear as small moving spots in a fluid medium. B)* E. coli *under 3000-fold magnification by a scanning electron microscope (J. T. Park, Tufts University School of Medicine). The rod shape is typical of this intestinal bacterium.*

Bacteria multiply by simple division, making a copy of their single chromosome and giving it to their progeny. Under the best laboratory conditions, growing in nutrient-rich media without competing predators, many types of bacteria can double their number within 20 minutes. In nature, they multiply less rapidly, often taking days to duplicate, since needed energy-producing materials are scarce and they are constantly in competition with neighboring microorganisms. For example, in the intestinal tract and on the skin, bacteria probably double no more than once every 12 to 24 hours. Although they can live as independent individual cells, they generally do not do so in nature. Instead, they exist in large numbers of colonies, each representing the progeny of a single cell, such as those seen on Koch's gelatin agar plates. As colonies, they live in the intestinal tract and on the skin. There they are referred to as our "intestinal flora" and "skin flora" or microbiota. They also reside on soil particles in natural soils and in the sludge at the bottom of lakes, streams, and oceans. As groups of individual living entities, bacteria work together in a microscopic society, like ants in their ant hills, to obtain nutrients for growth and for survival of their population against the competition of other bacteria and predatory microorganisms. In this way, bacteria can also be likened to animal cells that work together as an interactive unit in the body to perform a particular function, such as the cells making up our heart, kidneys, and liver.

A single bacterium does no damage in nature and has little chance of survival. It must produce a large number of progeny in order to have any impact. Millions of bacteria are needed to produce enough toxins to cause disease or to digest enough tissue to lead to destruction of our internal organs, such as the intestine, lungs, or liver. Billions of bacteria are needed in order for them to become a stable component of an ecosystem, be it a soil or water niche, and even more of them to become the predominant form of bacteria in that ecological niche. About 10^{14} (one hundred thousand billion) bacteria live on the skin and in the gut of a human being. This amount is about ten times more than all the tissue cells that make up an average 150-pound person. Thus, although not seen, bacteria represent a major component of our body.

Scientists distinguish individual bacteria by their shapes—some are spherical, some are rodlike—and by the way they stain with a particular chemical preparation called the Gram stain. Hans Christian Gram of Denmark discovered this method in the late 1880s. He saw a color difference among bacteria that were contaminating a tissue preparation that he had stained with specific dyes in order to look for damages to the tissue. He noted that, in some samples, bacteria became colored a deep purple by the stain and retained this color during washing. These were designated "stain positive." Others lost the stain and were able to be counterstained with another, lighter dye and were colored pink; these he called "stain negative." In a survey of all forms of bacteria, this simple staining process proved readily useful for identifying different bacteria and placing them into one of two groups. Today this method has remained a major way of distinguishing bacteria that are classified as either "gram-positive" or "gram-negative" (Table 2.1).

The Gram stain distinction derives from the differing composition of bacterial cell walls. Gram-negative bacteria, such as the common rod-shaped *Escherichia coli*, which are normal inhabitants of our guts, have a three-layer cell wall. The outer layer is made up of sugars attached to lipids; such a cell wall does not hold onto the Gram stain. The outer layer can be peeled away with appropriate dissolving agents, revealing a middle layer made mostly of protein. This middle layer maintains the cell's normal structure. Next to this layer is an inner layer, which, like the outer, is composed mostly of lipids and protein. The outer layer protects the cell against hazardous environmental materials, and the inner layer helps the bacterium to accumulate the materials it needs for energy and to excrete the materials that are toxic. Other common gram-negative bacteria are shaped like tiny spheres or cocci. These include the gonococcus and meningococcus, which can cause common infectious diseases.

22 The Antibiotic Paradox

Table 2.1. Bacteria and some common diseases.

Microorganisms	Common Name	Disease
Gram Stain Positive		
Streptococcus pneumoniae	Pneumococcus	Lobar (pneumococcal) pneumon Earache (otitis media), meningit
Streptococcus pyogenes	Strep "Flesh-eating" bacterium	Strep throat Necrotizing fasciitis
Staphylococcus aureus	Golden staph	Septicemia Skin boils
Entercoccus faecalis	Enterococcus	Septicemia
Gram Stain Negative		
Neisseria meningitidis	Meningococcus	Meningitis
Neisseria gonorrhoeae	Gonococcus	Gonorrhea
Hemophilus influenzae	H. flu	Earache (otitis media), meningit Pneumonia
Escherichia coli	Colibacillus	Urinary tract infection, septicem

The gram-positive bacteria include the rod-shaped soil bacilli, which are not associated with human disease, and the round-shaped streptococci and staphylococci, which live on the skin and in the mouth. These bacteria have only a single cell wall made up of a proteinlike material combined with a lipid. This layer allows the cells to hold on to the color in the Gram stain during washing. It is this single layer, like the inner layer of gram-negative bacteria, that performs the uptake and excretion functions necessary for cell viability (Figure 2.3).

As with all of us, bacteria need nutrients to survive. They live on simple environmental sources of the basic ingredients of matter—carbon, oxygen, hydrogen, and nitrogen. They obtain these by ingesting simple sugars located in the environment, by incorporating elements such as oxygen and nitrogen from the atmosphere into their diet, or by converting larger organic materials into needed substances. Some bacteria have special proteins, called enzymes, that can degrade organic matter into smaller nutritious elements. Others have the ability to break down complicated mixtures of fats or oils

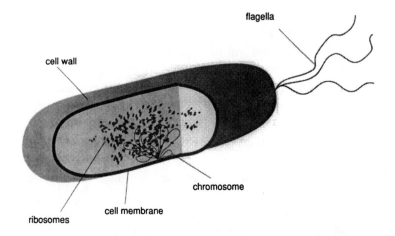

Figure 2.3. *Diagram of an E.* coli *bacterium and its major components. Note the multilayered exterior consisting of an inner cell membrane and an outer cell wall, a single DNA chromosome, flagella that help it move, and ribosomes, sites of protein synthesis (Bonnie Marshall, Tufts University School of Medicine).*

and live on the resultant enzymatically released nutrients. This is fortunate for us, since they are uniquely responsible for degrading organic wastes and for keeping our soils rich in nutrients for plant growth and agricultural products needed for human food production. They also can destroy toxic elements. The latter ability is presently being investigated as a future approach to the worldwide problem of environmental pollution. To help clean up toxic substances, bacteria that can degrade the harmful materials are being considered for purposeful release into polluted environments. An example is the use of "oil-eating" bacteria to help clean up the oil spill following the Exxon Valdez catastrophe in Alaska.

Among the many different kinds of bacteria existing in our environment, there are those capable of living only in the presence of air (aerobic) and only in the absence of air (anaerobic). Some can live under either condition. For instance, *E. coli*, which live outside in the environment as well as inside our intestinal tract, can survive and grow under aerobic or anaerobic conditions. On the other hand, *Clostridium botulinum*, the microorganism that releases the deadly toxin causing botulism, can survive only anaerobically. Air is toxic to this and other purely anaerobic microorganisms. Anaerobic bacteria are particularly active in compost pits, where they turn refuse into reusable nutrients for other living matter.

Bacteria are also an essential part of our digestive tract, where they, along with stomach and pancreatic juices, help to digest unabsorbed food residues as they move through our large intestines before their final exits in the excreta. This digestion releases important nutrients and vitamins needed for our growth and well-being that can then be absorbed from our intestines into our bodies. Bacteria line our skin with a protective coat of defense against invasion by more harmful varieties of microorganisms. In these and other ways, we rely on many varieties of bacteria to help us survive in the natural environment.

Bacteria and Disease

Bacteria can also be described on the basis of their ability to cause disease: those harmful to humans, animals, or plants are called "pathogenic," and those relatively harmless are designated "nonpathogenic." However, this designation must also include an understanding of the host involved, since the same bacteria may be harmless to humans, but harmful to other animals or plants, or vice versa. *Hemophilus influenzae* type b is a pathogen in humans, but not in animals. *Actinobacillus pleuropneumoniae* causes pneumonia in pigs, but not in mankind. *Salmonella typhi*, the cause of typhoid fever, is pathogenic only in humans. Other salmonellae can cause disease, chiefly diarrheas, in mankind and animals. The basis of pathogenicity is the ability of bacteria to cause an infection—a form of destruction of an organ. Normally, an infection requires from tens of thousands to millions of bacteria to generate disease.

Given these restraints, most bacteria entering our bodies by chance are quickly disarmed by our bodies' defenses and are unable to produce progeny. Among the most pathogenic bacteria, only 10 to 100 of them need to enter somewhere into our body to cause an infection. Disease occurs when bacteria multiply to high numbers before they can be removed or killed. Even one tubercle bacillus can cause tuberculosis if it enters and finds a protected site in the body of a susceptible person where it is able to multiply.

Each of us has natural defenses against bacterial invasion (Figure 2.4, next page). One of our major defense organs is the skin. A similar role is played by the mucous membranes that line our mouth, intestines, and outlets of the bladder and genital tracts. Mucus secretions bathe these cells, preventing bacteria from adhering to them. Some secretions even have antibacterial activity, such as lysozyme, found in tears. Cells lining our noses also contain threadlike hairs called cilia, which keep bacteria and other foreign objects from entering our upper respiratory passages and lungs.

If the skin is damaged, bacteria can enter through the break and then pass into the bloodstream, where they are disseminated to the rest of the body. Once past the skin, however, they face a second line of defense—circulating white blood cells ready to ingest and kill all invaders. The white cell response is helped by antibodies made against the invading organism. These antibodies help locate the foreign bacterium, attract white cell destroyers to it, or bring the organism to the spleen or lymph nodes, where it is destroyed. If the foreign invader can escape or overwhelm the white cells, it can grow to substantial enough numbers to cause real harm.

Some bacteria have intrinsic traits that can help them escape white cells. The composition of the bacterial outer cell wall is one of these. If it is rough or bulky in consistency, the bacterium is more easily engulfed by white blood cells. If it is smooth or slippery, however, the bacterium can evade the at-

Figure 2.4. *The human body has natural defenses against invasion by bacteria. These include the skin, mucous membranes lining the mouth and alimentary canal, cilia in the nasal passages, white blood cells, antibodies, and the reticuloendothelial system consisting of connective tissue cells that remove foreign objects, such as bacteria. They line the blood sinusoids of liver, spleen, bone marrow, and lymph channels in lymph nodes (Bonnie Marshall, Tufts University School of Medicine).*

tack and ingestion more easily, giving it a better chance to reach areas in the body where it can settle and multiply to sufficient numbers to cause disease. Other cell wall changes allow bacteria to avoid recognition by the white cells, or allow them to survive ingestion. To thwart the host defense more, some bacteria can actually survive and multiply *within* the white cell. Such is the case for the *Legionella* bacterium that causes the acute respiratory disease now known as Legionnaire's Disease. (It got its name from the epidemic of respiratory disease and deaths at the American Legion Convention in Philadelphia in 1976.) The bacterium *Mycobacterium tuberculosis*, which causes tuberculosis, also lives in cells, making it particularly difficult to treat. The bacteria causing plague and typhoid fever also live and reproduce in human cells. These kinds of microorganisms must be eliminated quickly from the body before they take up residence in the very defense systems designed to destroy them.

Another important trait carried by some pathogenic bacteria is the ability to attach and grow on the surface of tissue cells that make up the animal or plant being invaded. This "colonization" ability allows them to withstand the movement of bodily fluids, such as urine and feces. While attached to these cells, the bacteria take in nutrients released from the animal cells. These nutrients are necessary for survival of the attached bacteria and for the production of their offspring.

The unfavorable interactions of bacteria with our defense systems are enhanced when bacteria can synthesize substances toxic to human tissues. Such substances may be enzymes that can digest the walls of human cells to which they are attached, or they may be toxins that can rapidly kill the cells. Toxin-producing bacteria cause the uncomfortable and sometimes severe diarrhea we encounter when traveling to certain parts of the world. They are an unsuspected part of the food we eat there. So-called traveller's diarrhea is, in large part, caused by toxin-producing bacteria in uncooked foods that reach our intestinal tracts and produce the toxins that irritate and kill intestinal cells. Our intestinal tract responds by contracting vigorously, an action we know as cramps. There is typically a release of large amounts of fluid, as an attempt to eliminate the toxin and the toxin-producing bacteria. Eventually these bacterial invaders are lost or replaced by more acceptable, non-toxin-producing strains in the environment. Or, more favorably, we recover our own intestinal bacterial microbiota after we return home.

It may not seem logical that the local inhabitants don't chronically, or even periodically, suffer from these diarrhea-causing bacteria. Some do; but most do not. To some extent, these local people have established an intestinal flora that is adapted to the local bacteria and so they are less affected than are visitors who arrive bearing their own different flora. Local people also know what foods to avoid, something many visitors do not.

Scientifically, bacteria are only carrying out their own normal functions when they chance to find themselves inside an animal host. They have no purpose in invading, nor does invasion usually involve great numbers of bacteria. A few harmful bacteria may get into the body through a cut in the skin or a small opening in the mucous membranes. A few pathogens are ingested in foods, but most never get a hold on our bodies. Those intruding bacteria that escape detection and removal, however, thrive in excess nutrients. They form holes or abscesses in organs by releasing their destructive enzymes. We can most easily recognize this process when our body emits pus, which is a combination both of live and dead bacteria and of our own white cells that have arrived to destroy the bacteria.

The major energetic thrust of all microorganisms is to live and multiply. Yet should bacteria attack a vital organ—the heart, lung, or liver—they have ironically signed their own death warrants. In killing the person, the bacteria have, in fact, destroyed their life preserver and eventually die or are destroyed with the victim. This fatal and unwanted event differs dramatically from, say, a lion killing its prey for the food that will help it thrive. Microorganisms follow the biblical word to "live and multiply." Doing so, however, can lead to their own eventual demise.

Other Microorganisms

Many types of microscopic single-cell microorganisms exist in nature (Figure 2.5, next page). Some, such as those discussed already, are classified as bacteria because they are single-cell organisms and have no defined nuclei. Other examples of this type are the spirochetes and rickettsiae, which differ in size, shape, and genetic makeup from other bacteria. Taxonomists consider certain other single-cell microorganisms to be related more closely to animal and plant cells because they have a defined nucleus and other intracellular structures. These microorganisms include the yeasts, such as *Candida* or "monilia," and the fungi, which are of vastly different types. Only some of these are pathogenic to humans.

Viruses are much smaller than bacteria. Ten thousand of them can exist within a single cell. They are not independent microorganisms, but are dependent on the host cell in order to produce copies of themselves. They consist of genetic material, DNA or RNA, enveloped in a protein coat. They are specialized in the sense that they attach to a specific structure on the particular host cell. They then inject their single, small piece of nucleic acid, which interrupts the function of the cell. The cell either dies or becomes a factory in the production of thousands of copies of the virus. Virologists have identified a multitude of different viruses and many more are yet to be found. One virus causes the devastating disease AIDS; another causes warts; still another causes hepatitis (Figure 2.6, page 31). Others cause the common flu and winter cold.

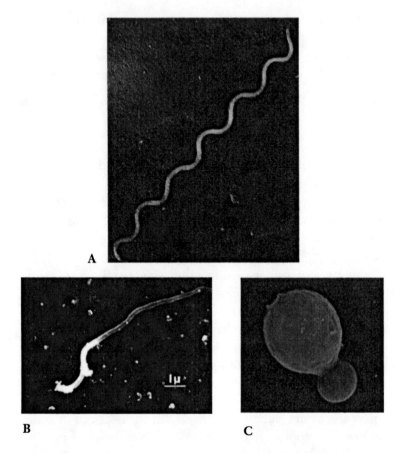

Figure 2.5. *Among microorganisms that exist in nature are bacteria, spirochetes, and yeast. Shown under scanning electron microscopy are: A) a spirochete called* Treponema pallidum, *which causes the venereal disease syphilis (magnified 1,300-fold) (James Miller, University of California, Los Angeles, California); B)* Borrelia bergendorfii, *a bacterium that causes Lyme disease (about 600-fold magnification) (Alan Steere, New England Medical Center, Boston); and C)* Candida albicans, *a common cause of yeast infection (magnified about 3500-fold) (David Soll, University of Iowa, Iowa City, Iowa).*

Figure 2.6. *Shown here by electron microscopy (about 37,500-fold magnification) are three viruses implicated in human diseases: A) the wart virus, which causes the common human wart; B) HIV–1, the virus that causes AIDS; and C) HHV–6, a herpes-like virus associated with the childhood disease "erythemum subitum" (Jay Levy, University of California, San Francisco).*

The origins and roles of these viruses in nature are unknown. Some biologists suggest that their existence results from random evolutionary events that produced agents capable of living on whole cells. In any case, they now contribute to the balance of nature. If a cell population increases, so do the viruses that kill these cells. Eventually, the cell population decreases, providing fewer hosts for the virus. Viruses without hosts are lost—and the balance in nature is restored.

A natural struggle continues between microorganisms (for instance, bacteria) and macroorganisms (for example, humans) and between microorganisms and other microorganisms. This conflict has taken place over the millennia in which bacteria have existed. Bacteria caused tuberculosis in ancient Egypt, as evidenced by scars and damaged tissues seen in mummies. Passages in the Bible refer to a venereal scourge, now known as gonorrhea, and evidence for this and another venereal disease, syphilis, has been found in ancient Egyptian tombs.

Our inherent ability to survive bacterial invasion rests on our natural defenses, namely, the production of antibodies and the activity of white cells. In the last half century, naturally occurring substances that aid in killing bacteria without harming the body have been added to these natural functions. These agents are the antibiotics.

Discovery of Antibiotics: Origins and Successes

With the acceptance of the germ theory of disease in the late 1800s came a change in the goals of treatment. An era began in which physicians and scientists searched for drugs that would kill the disease-causing agent, the bacterium or the parasite. The outcome of this search was the almost serendipitous discovery of antibiotics.

That living beings produce substances that inactivate or kill others was first put forth under the heading of "antibiosis" by the Frenchman Paul Vuillemin, head of Natural History at the medical faculty of the University of Nancy. His description, presented in 1889, dealt with negative effects or interactions that affected survival among animals and among plants, not among bacteria. He spoke of these as "influences antibiotiques," that is, "antibiotic influences." An antibiotic, as we now know it, is a natural substance made by one microorganism that inhibits growth of another microorganism. The actual term "antibiotic" is attributed to Selman Waksman, the American soil microbiologist and discoverer of the antibiotic streptomycin. He suggested the term in 1941 to the editor of *Biologic Abstracts* as a word for indexing a growing number of these kinds of antibacterial agents.

It would appear that antibiotics were inadvertently used even before their discovery. Ancient writings report the application of cloths impregnated with natural substances and other forms of organic matter onto wounds in order to help them heal. We suspect that these old remedies worked because they contained microorganisms producing antibiotics or the drugs themselves. Anthropologists have unearthed traces of the antibiotic tetracycline in thousand-year-old Nubian mummies. Microorganisms producing this antibiotic were found in soil samples that came from the same area where the mummies were discovered. Traces of tetracycline were recovered in grain as well. The Nubian nation survived a long time, from ancient times to the 14th century. Some scientists suggest that this long survival may in part be linked to the presence and use, either on purpose or by chance, of small amounts of crude antibiotics, such as the tetracyclines.

At the end of the 19th century, research scientists astutely put their energies into exploring methods that would use harmless bacteria to treat disease caused by harmful bacteria. Whole, harmless bacteria were fed to patients to compete

with the harmful disease-causing ones in hopes that the harmless ones would win out. In Paris in 1877, Louis Pasteur, with
his colleague Jules François Joubert, described how anthrax, a
disease caused by a bacillus, was suppressed in animals that
were injected with harmless soil bacteria. Ten years later, the
German scientist Rudolf Emmerich noted that guinea pigs
infected previously with a streptococcus were protected from
developing cholera when injected with the cholera bacillus.
He was the first to capitalize on this finding and use it to prevent cholera in animals.

About a year later in France, Charles Bouchard showed that
injection of small amounts of *Pseudomonas aeruginosa* protected rabbits from contracting anthrax. In related events,
other investigators noted that the typhoid fever bacillus survived longer when placed into sterile water than when introduced into water containing other organisms. All these findings implied a negative effect of the other bacteria on growth
of these pathogenic bacteria. The basis for these findings was
fully realized in retrospect only when antibiotics as products
of bacteria were discovered.

Historic developments that aided in identifying and enu-
merating bacteria contributed greatly to the discovery of antibiotics. Perhaps principal among these was Robert Koch's
gelatin-containing agar plate. Since investigators could grow
and count bacteria in the laboratory following a single day, or
night, of incubation, potential growth-inhibiting substances
could be tested in the agar along with bacteria. If the bacteria
grew, the substance was not active. If bacteria did not grow,
the substance was a potential agent for treating disease caused
by that bacterium.

The First Antibiotics

The first natural antibacterial product, that is, one that was
not made by chemists and thus merits the designation antibi-

otic, was pyocyanase, which rapidly gained international recognition. Its discovery in 1888 was partly serendipitous and partly the result of the search for these kinds of agents. E. de Freudenreich in Germany found that the blue pigment released in the broth culture of the blue-pus bacterium, *Bacillus pyocyaneus* (now known as *P. aeruginosa*), stopped the growth of other bacteria in the test tube. This activity suggested that the bacteria were producing a potentially useful agent to treat human disease caused by bacteria susceptible to this material.

Rudolf Emmerich, who had previously focused on microbe-microbe interactions, joined with Oscar Loew, also from Germany, to investigate this phenomenon further. They confirmed the previous findings and named the substance "pyocyanase" after the producing bacterium, adding "ase" because they considered the activity to be that of an enzyme protein. (It was shown later to be made of a lipid.) They performed the first extensive clinical trials of pyocyanase in 1889. Their reports lauded the beneficial effects of the drug not only in inhibiting bacterial growth but also in actually killing pathogenic bacteria, including those causing typhoid fever, anthrax, diphtheria, plague, and skin abscesses. The discovery was followed with great interest and excitement since it heralded a major breakthrough. When it came to applying these laboratory results to the patient, however, pyocyanase lost its luster. It was toxic and unstable. It was not the lifesaving potion they had sought. Still, its use persisted for almost thirty years, mainly as a topical ointment on the skin. By 1913, reports about any therapeutic efficacy of pyocyanase had almost disappeared.

Paul Ehrlich, a chemist working in Berlin, took a different approach. He was fascinated by dyes that stained tissues and microorganisms. He reasoned that such selectivity could help find a "magic bullet," that is, a substance that rids the body selectively of the infecting microorganism, whether it be a bacterium or parasite, without harming the body tissues. His first

36   The Antibiotic Paradox

successful candidate product, reported in 1910, was the drug Salvarsan, a chemical dye linked to arsenic. Its discovery came out of his search for agents to treat the trypanosome parasite that causes African sleeping sickness. Salvarsan received its greatest recognition when it was shown to help patients afflicted with syphilis. The drug worked, but not uniformly, and the toxicity of the arsenic derivative subjected patients to severe and sometimes painful and debilitating side effects. Still, it was a breakthrough—the first direct treatment of this common disease. Its discovery opened the door to a new era of interest in chemotherapy.

The early decades of the 20th century passed, however, without much advancement in the search for antibacterial substances. It is believed that the failure of pyocyanase and other candidates to live up to Ehrlich's "magic bullet" dream probably had a discouraging effect on the search for other compounds of this type. Reports surfaced of better antiseptics—agents that would sterilize surgical instruments and even certain skin wounds—but these could not be taken into the body. Many of these could not even be used on humans because they were toxic to the skin. Instead, they were relegated to disinfecting utensils, such as those used in surgery. None of these materials proved to be that magic substance that would be effective and nontoxic when taken internally. General enthusiasm for the ideal substance waned.

Discovery of Penicillin

Still, some laboratories persisted in the search. Alexander Fleming, working at St. Mary's Hospital in London, discovered and reported in the 1920s a naturally occurring antibacterial substance in human tears that caused certain bacterial cells to break open and die. He called this material "lysozyme," since it caused susceptible bacteria to fall apart, or to lyse. Unfortunately, it too proved to have no practical place as a therapeutic agent. For one, its effectiveness was mostly limited to nonpathogenic bacteria and, additionally, it was not easily made in large enough amounts to allow for sufficient testing in people or animals. Its importance lay more in its being one of the first natural substances identified within humans with the real or potential role of protecting us against bacterial invasion.

In 1928, Fleming happened on his second antibacterial discovery—this time a major one. Coming back from a weekend vacation, he went through his usual routine of looking at some of the old plates that had been left in his work area. In doing so, he noticed a discarded plate that had not yet been submerged in a detergent solution. There he saw that colonies of the common skin organism *Staphylococcus* had lysed—fallen apart—seemingly by the product of a mold growing in the adjacent area. He observed that the lysis occurred only in this one area and noted that this effect was apparently caused by the mold that was growing next to the bacterial colonies on the plate (Figure 2.7, next page). Had this gelatin plate been submerged into the detergent solution along with all the others, which was the case for the majority of discarded plates, this history-making discovery would not have been made, at least not then.

As Fleming freely admitted, the interference with bacterial growth by a fungus had been seen by many others before him, but no one had paid much attention to the phenomenon. In the late 1890s, a professor at Johns Hopkins University in Baltimore had reportedly showed his students an agar plate on which a mold appeared to be inhibiting the growth of bacteria isolated from urine. But the significance of this observation was not appreciated—at least there was no apparent follow-up of the finding. An Italian researcher from Naples, Vincenzo Tiberio, publishing in Italian in 1895, had described in some detail natural substances, extracted from molds, with antibacterial activities resembling penicillin.[1] Clearly, Fleming knew nothing about these reports. But in retrospect, they preceded Fleming's findings by thirty years, and were also those of serendipity and observation.

Fleming was fascinated by the phenomenon and guessed that he was witnessing a medically important event, the actual falling apart, or lysis, of already-formed colonies (Figure 2.8, page 40).

Perhaps this also reminded him of his work on lysozyme, which also caused lysis, although lysozyme's effect was on individual bacteria rather than on whole colonies. Being familiar with one kind of lytic agent, he happened upon another. This one came not from human fluids but was presumably made by the mold on the plate. Fleming soon demonstrated that, in fact, the mold made a substance small enough to diffuse through the agar and lyse the bacteria. He called it "penicillin" after the *Penicillium* mold that had produced it. By extracting the substance from cultures of the mold, he was able to show its antibacterial activity directly. Penicillin was so uniquely active that small amounts of culture fluids could produce this killing effect. And, more importantly, it triumphed over a very common and deadly bacterium, *Staphylococcus aureus*, which caused skin infections, often leading to bloodborne dangerous septic disease. The events surrounding Fleming's discovery have challenged historians and microbiologists trying to reproduce the exact conditions that led to his seeing this lytic event on the agar plates. Still, the proof of the happening lies in the dried original plate, which Fleming kept and which remains in the archives at St. Mary's Hospital in London.

Penicillium mold

full-grown colonies

lysed staphylococcal colonies

Figure 2.7. *Diagram of the original plate observed by Alexander Fleming in 1928 showing lysis of staphylococcal colonies growing near a mold that happened to be on the same plate (Bonnie Marshall, Tufts University School of Medicine).*

Prontosil: Revival of Interest in Antibiotics

Fleming is credited with discovering our first true antibiotic, penicillin. While the discovery was made in 1928, use of penicillin as a therapeutic agent to treat infections in humans did not occur until the 1940s. Fleming attributed this delay to a lack of biochemical and microbiological expertise at the time. There also existed at that time a mentality that discouraged the possibility of finding substances that could be used internally to treat major infectious diseases. As we mentioned before, this lack of initiative was probably the legacy of the fail-

Figure 2.8. *Alexander Fleming (1881–1955), who discovered penicillin in 1928 (G. MacFarlane,* Alexander Fleming: The Man and the Myth, *Harvard University Press, Cambridge. Reprinted by permission).*

ure of pyocyanase and the toxicity of Salvarsan. But an event in the 1930s turned this attitude around.

Gerhard Domagk, director of research at I. G. Farbenindustrie in Germany, was examining different chemical dyes for their effect on bacterial infections. In the course of these studies, he discovered an antibacterial agent that worked when given to animals. This was not an antibiotic in the true sense of the word, since it was man-made and not a natural product. Like penicillin, its discovery occurred somewhat by accident. Domagk found that Prontosil, a newly patented dye, cured diseases caused by the streptococcus bacteria when injected into diseased mice. He had been motivated to try dyes as antimicrobials because he knew that they stained bacteria as well as tissues, and he reasoned that perhaps, when taken up by the bacteria, they would interfere with growth. It is interesting to note that Domagk and colleagues tested all the chemicals, including Prontosil, in animals as well as test tubes. Had he relied only on the test tube assay, his discovery would never have been made.

Prontosil was active only when put into mice and not when tested against growing bacteria in a test tube—an unusual finding not observed for any other previously described agent. The answer to this mystery came later. Others discovered that it was not the dye part of the molecule but the chemical attached to it, the sulfonamide portion, that, when released during metabolism of the compound in the body, killed the bacteria.

It was the effectiveness of Prontosil, and later other sulfonamide derivatives, that scientists regard as the critical event leading to the resurgence of interest in antibiotics. At long last, physicians had an agent that, when taken internally, worked and was nontoxic and stable. The disappointing results of pyocyanase and other ineffective agents were relegated to ancient history. This discovery created a new receptive atmosphere for the development and production of penicillin, which had already been discovered seven years before Domagk's eventful experiments with Prontosil. There was renewed interest in discovering other "magic bullets." Some were to be newly discovered; other potential agents were being reexamined in a new, more optimistic light.

The Search for Antibiotics

With the successes of sulfonamides known widely, the quest for other forms of antibacterial agents revived. Common soil dug up from anywhere in the ground became the focus of these new searches. As far back as the 1890s, Robert Koch, the inventor of the gelatin plate, was fascinated by the fact that pathogenic bacteria died when put into soil. He wondered why. A half century later, in the 1940s, Selman Waksman and other soil microbiologists went back to examine the same phenomenon. They searched in hopes of finding the inhibitors of bacterial growth in the soil, notably among the soil microorganisms themselves.

Waksman said at a meeting of the National Academy of Sciences in Washington in 1940:

> Bacteria pathogenic to man and animals find their way to the soil, either in the excreta of the hosts or in their remains. If one considers the period for which animals and plants have existed on this planet and the great numbers of disease-producing microbes that must have thus gained entrance into the soil, one can only wonder that the soil harbors so few bacteria capable of causing infectious diseases in man and animals. . . . It was suggested that the cause of the disappearance of these disease-producing organisms in the soil is to be looked for among the soil-inhabiting microbes, antagonistic to the pathogens and bringing about their rapid destruction in the soil.[2]

On the basis of these considerations, Waksman and others went to the soil, "panning" for these antagonistic substances. Their work did not go unrewarded. Their activities not only advanced the science of soil microbiology but also led to the golden age of antibiotic discovery.

Waksman's suppositions and interpretations in the 1940s grew out of a long period of experiments in soil microbiology that he had begun several decades before. This initial work had focused on the discovery of bacteria as sources of enzymes for chemical processes. His new efforts once again generated great interest in the soil for different kinds of substances, namely, those that could cure infections.

Therefore, it is perhaps not surprising that one of Waksman's former students, René J. Dubos, a graduate of the French National Institute of Agronomy in Paris who had worked with Waksman on his prior research, turned to the soil in his search for antibiotics. In 1939, while at the Rockefeller Institute, Dubos isolated, for the first time, an antibiotic-producing soil microorganism. His discovery also led to the first clinically useful antibiotic, beating the discovery of penicillin by about five years. By mixing the infectious bacteria *Staphylococcus* with cultures of different soil bacteria, Dubos noticed one culture that would not allow growth of the staphylococci. In this successful culture, he identified a *Bacillus brevis* bacterium that excreted a substance into the culture fluid that killed the staphylococci. Because this substance only seemed to kill the gram-positive organisms—that group of bacteria identified by their ability to take up the stain developed by Gram—Dubos named it "gramicidin." He presented his discovery to the world at the International Congress of Microbiology in New York in 1940. Following on the heels of the synthetic sulfonamides, gramicidin was the first natural product extracted from a soil organism and shown to have these antibacterial properties. But the drug had certain major drawbacks, in particular, a severe toxicity when given intravenously. Still, gramicidin found a place in human therapy as an external application for minor skin infections, a purpose for which it is still used today.

Development of Penicillin

On the other side of the Atlantic, a team led by the English pathologist Howard Florey was responsible for the renewed interest in finding more antibiotics. Encouraged by the successes of sulfonamides, Florey decided to put together a team to evaluate antibacterials. He was soon joined by Ernst Chain, a German-born biochemist with whom he would collaborate for years. They began their experiments in the late 1930s and continued into the fifth decade. After a search of the literature for potential substances, they decided to begin with lysozyme. But after several years they realized that this was not the agent to be pursued. They moved to another of Fleming's agents, penicillin. They were working in Oxford, not far from London, where Fleming was still located at St. Mary's Hospital. While Fleming had continued to work on penicillin, he was not able to purify enough of it to test in animals or humans.

For penicillin, then, it was Florey and Chain who became the clear flag bearers. They and their colleagues learned how to extract the substance, how to keep it stable, and how to produce it in amounts sufficient to test in animals. Their results were spectacular. Mice destined to die from infection were miraculously cured by this drug. When sufficient quantities were made to test in people, the limited amounts available were used only on very sick patients whose infectious disease had reached near fatal proportions. Use of even very small amounts of penicillin, in a crude state, was able to turn the tide of the infection and cure individuals considered to be on their death beds. In some instances, the drug was so scarce that any of it that came out in the patients' urine was reextracted and used for subsequent doses!

The small amounts of penicillin were only enough to treat a limited number of patients; however, joint efforts by Florey and his colleagues, along with American physicians and scientists, as well as the trials following the Cocoanut Grove fire, convinced United States pharmaceutical firms and the United States government to begin producing it in large quantities. Using an unusual form of intraindustry cooperation, several companies accelerated the scale of production. Initially, penicillin was reserved exclusively to treat soldiers and a few lucky civilians. It more or less "belonged" to the military. Eventually, by 1944, penicillin became available to the public. With its widespread use came more publicity, this time, staggering. Fleming was called "one of the great scientists of the 20th century." His picture was featured on the May 15, 1944, cover of *Time* magazine. Without the revelatory power of television, with only newsreels, radio, and newspapers, the thrilling story of the miracle of penicillin was told and retold to audiences around the world.

Soon, the discovery of penicillin took on mythic proportions. It was as if Prometheus had stolen fire from the gods. The applications of this wonder drug seemed all but limitless. In fact, people began to assume that it could cure and help any disease. Even within the medical literature of the time, we can find passages stating that penicillin had worked on cancers and on viral infections—diseases and conditions on which we now know penicillin has no effect. These distorted expectations became a part of the mystique surrounding penicillin and other antibiotics, which has been carried over even into present times. To many, an antibiotic is a "cure-all" to be taken for any illness, though, in fact, it can treat only certain illnesses. In the 1940s there was no way to control what was being said or thought about penicillin. Penicillin became whatever people wanted it to be. Faced with the ravages of war, people needed something to pin their hopes on. To some degree, penicillin played that role and public consensus mandated that the drug be available to everyone.

Streptomycin: A Cure for Tuberculosis

The first major finding in the search for an internally useful antibiotic from soil was made in 1943 by Selman Waksman and his group working at the New Jersey State Agriculture Experimental Station at Rutgers University. Aware of the discovery of gramicidin by Dubos, Waksman had already turned his attention away from enzymes produced by soil bacteria and began to look for those making antibiotics. From over 10,000 cultures of potential producers, Waksman and his colleagues, in collaboration with Merck and Company in nearby Rahway, New Jersey, selected ten microorganisms that seemed to hold the most promise. Among these was *Streptomyces griseus*. This producer proved to be different from any of the microorganisms previously found to make antibiotics. It was neither a mold nor a member of the *Bacillus* group of bacteria, such as the one that made gramicidin. It was a member of another family of soil bacteria, the actinomycetes. The antibiotic that *S. griseus* produced was subsequently called "streptomycin."

Streptomycin proved effective not only in the test tube, but also in people. It was active against bacteria that caused common infections, such as urinary tract infections, and against those causing meningitis; it also was effective in combatting more unusual ones, like the systemic disease tularemia, which is spread by infected animals and ticks. Yet its most acclaimed use was discovered when it was found to kill the then untouchable bacterium *Mycobacterium tuberculosis*, the cause of tuberculosis. This was the first antibiotic or drug of any kind that offered hope to victims suffering from this chronic, debilitating, and often fatal disease.

Streptomycin, however, triggered certain side effects that were not observed with penicillin. Streptomycin, in the accumulated dosage needed to cure the disease, could cause damage to the kidneys and lead to temporary and even persistent deafness. Attempts to modify it chemically in order to reduce its toxicity were not successful. A second problem proved to be even more critical, namely, that during therapy, bacteria became resistant to the killing effect of streptomycin at a frequency that compromised treatment. This phenomenon did not occur very easily with the antibiotics penicillin or gramicidin. Although penicillin-resistant bacteria existed, their numbers were small and they did not pose a great clinical dilemma. Mutants did not appear during drug therapy as they did with streptomycin.

The rapid emergence of mutants resistant to streptomycin encouraged the Merck laboratories and other groups to look for other antibiotics that were safer than streptomycin and to which spontaneous resistance was less likely to occur. The fruit of these efforts was the antibiotic neomycin, to which bacteria did not develop resistance so easily. The drug was also very toxic, however. It is used today primarily in topical antibacterial ointments. Neomycin is related structurally to streptomycin and became the second in this "aminoglycoside" group of antibiotics, to which were later added the antibiotics kanamycin (1957), gentamicin (1963), tobramycin (1971), and amikacin (1976), a semisynthetic derivative of kanamycin. These latter antibiotics have proven very useful as systemic treatment agents.

The Birth of Broad-Spectrum Agents

Chloramphenicol

Other drugs still in use today also made their appearance at the end of the 1940s. A Yale University microbiologist, Paul Burkholder, was conducting his own search for antibiotic-producing microorganisms in soils that he had obtained from many different countries. When he found microorganisms that produced substances that inhibited the growth of other bacteria, he would send them to the Parke Davis Company in Detroit for confirmation and additional testing. In the summer of 1947, he discovered one microorganism, from a soil sample collected in a field in Caracas, Venezuela, that produced an inhibitory substance that appeared to kill a wide variety of bacterial types. The diversity of bacteria affected made the discovery exciting and novel. Burkholder extended his studies with the microorganism to more and more different kinds of bacteria and found that the drug was the first discovered that inhibited both gram-positive and gram-negative bacteria, that is, bacteria with very different cell wall structures as distinguished by the Gram stain. The compound was named *Chloromycetin*, based on the fact that it contained a chlorine atom (chloro) and was produced by a member of the actinomycete (mycin) family (later named *Streptomyces venezuelae* after its country of origin).

Chloromycetin, also known as the chemical substance chloramphenicol, rose to prominence when investigators discovered that its spectrum of activity included members of a different type of bacterial group, the rickettsiae. These infectious agents, carried by ticks and other mites, cause epidemic typhus and Rocky Mountain Spotted Fever, both potentially fatal diseases. The first human trial of chloramphenicol came in La Paz, Bolivia, where public health officials were trying to cope with an epidemic of typhus. Parke Davis sent down as much of the chloramphenicol as they could. Fourteen of the fifty patients for whom there was no chloramphenicol died, but all twenty-two who were treated recovered.

Having identified both a new antibiotic and the cure of a previously untreatable disease, investigators went on to test the effect of the drug against other bacteria. They found that chloramphenicol was also very effective in the treatment of the bacterium that causes typhoid fever. These bacteria were not susceptible to any antibiotic known at the time.

The success of chloramphenicol, however, was marred by the discovery that the drug had potentially life-threatening toxic side effects. A small percentage of treated patients (now known to be about one in 40,000) suffered from bone marrow suppression, causing the loss of circulating red cells and white cells. A smaller number went on to irreversible total bone marrow collapse leading to anemias and even leukemias. As a consequence, the United States and other countries decided it was too risky to keep chloramphenicol as a first-line therapy for any disease. In special instances it is still used today, notably for serious illnesses that have not responded to other antibiotics. In the developing world, however, despite its toxicity, chloramphenicol is used extensively to treat severe diarrheas and pneumonias. This practice continues because the drug is so inexpensive and, therefore, more easily affordable in areas where the cost of substitute drugs precludes their widespread use. Another rationale for its use would be the suspicion that the patient with diarrhea could have typhoid fever, for which chloramphenicol has been a drug of choice. Today, however, strains causing this disease are resistant to this drug and many others, as we shall discuss later.

The Tetracyclines

Chloramphenicol was the first of the class of "broad-spectrum" antibiotics. Its reserved use, because of toxicity, was probably facilitated by the finding of other antibiotics with wide antimicrobial activity.

At the same time that Burkholder was studying chloramphenicol, Benjamin Duggar, at the Lederle Laboratories in Pearl River, New York, became fascinated by a microorganism that excreted a golden-colored substance that had novel antibiotic properties. The microorganism, now called *Streptomyces aureofaciens*, produced the antibiotic then called aureomycin and now known as chlortetracycline, the first member of the tetracycline family of antibiotics. The drug, introduced in 1948, showed low toxicity and a broad spectrum of activity against bacteria. Both features propelled it to worldwide use within one to two years of its introduction into the clinical arena. It also proved effective against rickettsiae and the typhoid bacillus as well as a long list of other disease-causing bacteria, making it a clear alternative to the more toxic chloramphenicol. By 1955, only seven years after chlortetracycline was introduced, over 8,000 papers were already published describing its use in both acute and chronic infections.

Its eventual low price and broad spectrum of activity have made it a commonly used antibiotic in the developing world. Today tetracyclines rank second only to penicillins in world production and world use.

Following the discovery of these first-generation antibiotics, more antibiotics were discovered, tested, and introduced with unprecedented rapidity. These events occurred in countries all over the world, notably during the decades of the 1950s, 1960s, and early 1970s (Table 2.2).

The Cephalosporins: Other Penicillin-Like Antibiotics with Broad-Spectrum Activity

Two unique penicillin-like drugs, cephalothin and cephaloridine, were introduced in 1964. The time from discovery to entry into the clinical arena was much longer than with previous antibiotics. The initial discovery leading to the development of these drugs came in 1945 by the Italian microbiologist Giuseppe Brotsu. He noticed antibacterial activity in extracts from a mold he found in a sewer outlet off the coast of Sardinia. It took years to purify the active agent. He sent his materials to Florey and researchers at Oxford, who found a number of different antibiotics in the culture fluid. Once the chemical structure of the most active component was known, derivatives that were more stable and retained high and broad-spectrum antibacterial activity were made. The two cephalosporins mentioned above were the fruits of these efforts. Three years later, in 1967, two orally effective cephalosporins were ready for clinical use. Continued modification of cephalosporins, as with penicillins, has led to more and more derivatives with properties varying in rate and extent of oral absorption, length of time in the body, spectrum of activity, and insensitivity to cephalosporin-degrading enzymes, the so-called cephalosporinases.

Table 2.2. Chronology of antimicrobial discovery and clinical use (1929–2000).

	Event	Country
1929	penicillin discovered	England
1932	sulfonamides (Prontosil) discovered	Germany
1939	gramicidin discovered	United States
1942	penicillin introduced	England and United States
1943	streptomycin discovered	United States
1943	bacitracin discovered	United States
1945	cephalosporins discovered	Italy
1947	chloramphenicol discovered	United States
1947	chlortetracycline discovered	United States
1949	neomycin discovered	United States
1950	oxytetracycline discovered	United States
1952	erythromycin discovered	United States
1956	vancomycin discovered	United States
1957	kanamycin discovered	Japan
1960	methicillin introduced	England and United States
1961	ampicillin introduced	England
1961	spectinomycin reported	United States
1963	gentamicin discovered	United States
1964	cephalosporins introduced	England
1964	vancomycin introduced	United States
1966	doxycycline introduced	United States
1967	clindamycin reported	United States
1971	rifampicin introduced	United States
1971	tobramycin discovered	United States
1972	cephamycins (cefoxitin) discovered	United States
1972	minocycline introduced	United States
1974	cotrimoxazole introduced	United States
1976	amikacin introduced	United States
1984	amoxicillin/clavulanate introduced	United States and Europe
1987	imipenem/cilastin introduced	United States
1987	ciprofloxacin introduced	United States and Europe
1993	azithromycin and clarithromycin introduced	United States
1999	quinupristin/dalfopristin introduced	United States
2000	linezolid introduced	United States

Synthesis of Methicillin in Response to Mounting Penicillin Resistance

Early in the antibiotic era, with the advent of oral and other noninjectible forms of penicillin, this valued agent began to be used in a large variety of over-the-counter preparations, including "salves, throat lozenges, nasal ointments, and even cosmetic creams"—all "marketed in response to the public clamor for the 'miracle drug'."[3]

By 1955, most countries restricted the use of penicillin to that by prescription only. But widespread usage had already occurred. This uncontrolled early usage led to a legacy of growing resistance in that decade and beyond, a widespread resistance to penicillin, especially among the staphylococci. Historically, a concerted effort was made by pharmaceutical houses to deal with this resistance, to try to circumvent the enzymatic degradation of this valued therapeutic agent.

An answer to the resistance problem came with the discovery and introduction of methicillin in the early 1960s. This semisynthetic penicillin was insensitive to the bacterial enzymes that degraded penicillin. Other derivatives able to be taken orally soon followed. While this advance initially stemmed the avalanche of penicillin resistance, it revealed yet another unwelcomed surprise—bacterial resistance to this semisynthetic drug itself, a problem now faced worldwide.

The Synthetic Antimicrobials

Added to the growing field of naturally occurring antibacterial substances were substances that were chemically synthesized. The first group of these was the sulfonamide family, whose successful use preceded all of the "natural" antibiotics. As effective as antibiotics are, these products were not naturally produced by other bacteria and consequently have been called synthetic antimicrobials, or just antimicrobials. Sulfonamide derivatives followed the discovery that the active antibacterial agent in Prontosil was in actuality a sulfonamide. These were synthesized in the 1930s and into the 1940s in many different forms, enlarging their spectrum of activity, their pharmacologic features (that is, the length of time they would reside in the body), and the method of inoculation, whether by injection or by mouth. The development of this group of highly effective drugs forms the foundation of this era of antimicrobial discovery and development. Today, sulfonamides still represent a relatively large proportion of all antimicrobial agents being produced and sold throughout the world.

Trimethoprim was the second of the synthetic antimicrobials to take its place in the popular marketplace. Its introduction in the 1970s came in combination with a sulfonamide, sulfamethoxazole, in a single medication form called cotrimoxazole, for the treatment of gram-negative and gram-positive infections. It proved extremely effective against infectious microorganisms of the urinary tract and in systemic infections, such as those caused by *Salmonella*, *E. coli*, or *Hemophilus*. Its ability to penetrate deeply into tissues made it an alternative for the therapy of such diseases as typhoid fever, where the bacteria often "hide" in the gallbladder or within lymph nodes. The combination of trimethoprim and a sulfonamide was touted and advanced because it involved the use of two agents, both synthetic, and both of which acted on naturally occurring enzymes at different steps in a metabolic pathway essential to the growth of bacteria. It was assumed that resistance to two synthetic agents would not appear. That assumption may have held, had sulfonamide resistance not been already so prominent when this drug was introduced. In fact, it was shown that the high success rate of the combination drug was essentially linked to the trimethoprim itself. In a departure from the usual mode of introduction, trimethoprim, as a therapeutic alone, was introduced later, after it had already been used in combination with a sulfonamide.

Recently, another group of synthetic agents has taken center stage. These drugs are related to an older synthetic agent, nalidixic acid. They have proven effective against a wide variety of gram-positive and gram-negative bacteria. The core of these agents is a chemical structure called a "quinolone," to which a fluorine atom was added and thus they are called fluoroquinolones. In contrast to the rapid emergence of bacteria resistant to nalidixic acid, in a frequency resembling that of streptomycin, these new agents showed an exceedingly lower tendency to select resistant mutants.

The fluoroquinolones can be taken by mouth and still achieve a high concentration in the blood stream. This feature permits excellent antibacterial coverage by the medication when taken at home, an advantage in this day of rising hospital costs. The fluoroquinolones are, in fact, being used as agents for treatment of infectious diseases that require prolonged therapy of anywhere from several weeks to several months.

Given these advantages, that is, low toxicity and infrequent selection of resistant mutants, fluoroquinolones became a popular new group of antimicrobial agents. More and more derivatives have appeared, and additional ones are still coming onto the market. Each derivative differs from the others in its time of circulation in the body and the group of microorganisms on which it is active. For instance, some derivatives have shown surprising efficacy against bacteria that have been traditionally difficult to treat, such as the bacteria causing leprosy.

Sales of fluoroquinolones soared in the aftermath of resistance to other antibiotics. The most successful member was ciprofloxacin, for which sales were over $1 billion annually by the end of the 1990s. Still, despite difficulty in selecting resistant mutants in the laboratory, the increasing use of these agents, particularly in the community, led to a variety of highly resistant bacterial strains, which totally thwarted their activity—surprising the producers and clinicians. Staphylococci, particularly the threatening methicillin-resistant variety, MRSA, appeared almost "overnight" with high-level fluoroquinolone resistance accompanying its many other drug resistances. One recent study even correlated the risk of contracting MRSA with the use of fluoroquinolones by the patient.

Thus, despite highly effective activity and difficulty in selecting resistant mutants in the laboratory, the fluoroquinolones, like other antibiotics, fell victim to overuse and misuse, namely, the emergence of strains no longer susceptible to them.

Attacking Resistance Directly

Another way around resistance was evident in drug combinations appearing through the 1980s and 1990s that included an inhibition of the enzymes that degraded penicillins. The first to show this activity, clavulanic acid, then sulbactam, and finally tazobactam were combined with a penicillin to restore the activity of the penicillin partner. The first combination and most successful of these was *Augmentin*, introduced by Beecham Pharmaceuticals, which combined clavulanic acid with amoxicillin. Clavulanic acid's disarming of the penicillin-destructive enzyme allowed amoxicillin to do its job. The combination product joined safety with efficacy and pioneered the notion that once known, resistance mechanisms could be directly attacked, leading to a new man-made antibiotic.

The Future of Antibiotics

It is only in the past half century that we have seen the rapid development and production of antibiotics. In 1949, the United States produced penicillin and streptomycin at a rate of 6.5 tons per month. In 1954, between 400,000 and 500,000 pounds of broad-spectrum antibiotics were being made. Today, the United States produces an estimated 50 million pounds annually. How much of this amount is provided in the U.S. as opposed to sold elsewhere is not certain, but most agree it is between 75–85%. This figure alone tells us something about the growth of this industry.

The quest for new antibiotics continues, but at a slower pace. New drug discoveries too often come up with an antibiotic that is not really original, but is a derivative member of a family already described. Chemical synthesis to modify antibiotics already in hand offers some approach to developing derivatives that are truly different.

At the very end of the 1990s and the beginning of the year 2000, two new antibiotics were approved for use in the United States and elsewhere. One was a combination of streptogramins (quinupristin/dalfopristin) developed by Rhone-Polenc Rorer and sold under the name *Synercid*. It inhibits growth of gram-positive bacteria, including MRSA. The other new drug, called linezolid or *Zyvox* and introduced by Pharmacia, also provides only gram-positive activity. Of note, *Zyvox* is the first structurally new antibiotic in the past 25–30 years. Since the structurally related streptogramins have already been used for years as an animal growth promoter called virginiamycin, resistance to *Synercid* was not difficult to find among certain bacteria from animals that received it. More recently, strains of enterococci and *Staphylococcus aureus* resistant to linezolid have emerged during long-term treatments. The unwanted appearance of resistant strains in people being treated with these new drugs undermines their hoped-for, long-term efficacy and urges careful use to avoid an increased resistance problem. It is clear, however, that more initiatives to identify truly new antibiotics, and especially to safeguard the antibiotics we now have, are the goals for the next decade.

chapter three

Reliance on Medicines and Self-Medication

The Seeds of Antibiotic Misuse

Antibiotics are a medical treasure, perhaps the most important therapeutic discovery in the history of medicine. But they are being misused. In some cases, they are taken when they are not needed at all; in others, they are prescribed and used inappropriately. For example, they are given in too small or too large amounts or for too long or too short periods of time. The old adage applies here. "Too much of a good thing can be bad." In the case of antibiotics, we must add, "so can too little." Not only quantity, but length of usage, either too long or too short, can affect the therapeutic and environmental consequences of these agents.

Misuse has led to the decreased effectiveness of antibiotics because of the emergence of bacteria that are resistant to them. Antibiotics, like other pharmaceuticals, "suffer" from the present-day reliance on medication to cure every ailment, the "pill for every ill" belief. In the quest for a rapid relief of symptoms, medicines that are freely available to people are being misused. So it is with antibiotics. They have been overused and used inappropriately, creating in their wake an environment where antibiotic-resistant bacteria survive.

Overreliance on medicine to treat an array of illnesses is not unique to antibiotics. It reflects humanity's understandable desire for relief from illness, the rush to use medicines in order to return to a normal daily life. This attitude, however, was not always so prominent. In early times, when medicinal substances were not plentiful, the power of the word and communication with the spirits played an important role. The inclusion of a nonmedicinal approach to therapy was retained for a long time during and after the discovery of effective medications. Eventually, however, the chant and the communication were replaced almost completely by medicines.

Historical Overview

A brief account of the history leading to modern-day medicine is worth noting, since it sets the background in which antibiotics were discovered and may help to explain society's current expectations and attitudes toward these drugs.

Early ancestors believed that each and every distinct "thing"—whether a tree, a stone, or a drinking vessel—was imbued with a spirit. When someone suddenly fell ill, it was assumed that an object was taking vengeance for a slight or grievance that had been committed against it—an unacceptable offering, a felled tree, an overturned stone. Suffering from headache, fever, stomach cramps, or aching muscles, the patient would seek out a healer to calm the spirits and dispel the symptoms. This healer, whether self-proclaimed or appointed, would proceed, as he and his forebears had done many times before, to address the "souls in conflict" and, thereby, cure the illness. The healer returned the patient and the object to a proper balance or relationship.

The healer believed he communicated with and appeased the spirits through his invocations. Some healers made cuts in the body to let blood or pus run out—to encourage the evil spirit to leave. Sacrifices or offerings were often made to the gods to abate their anger. In very early times, it was the voice of the healer and his accepted, even magical, powers that were valued even above those of the natural substances that accompanied the ritual.

That nonmedicinal approaches worked attests to the power of suggestion that can mobilize processes in our own body and help relieve symptoms. Today, we call this the "placebo effect"—the relief of disease or symptoms caused by the mere suggestion that the medication will work and that the person will get better. The "placebo effect" is that force or reaction that influences disease via changes in the body in response to positive feelings about treatment. In testing the efficacy of a drug, contemporary clinical researchers always give a placebo, usually a sugar or chalk pill, to half the patients in the test while the other half receives the real medication. Even the doctors giving out the drug do not know which pill they are dispensing. If the drug shows a statistically-higher benefit over the placebo, then it is considered truly therapeutic. It has demonstrated its potency. While yet to be fully understood, the placebo effect may be linked to products that the cells of our bodies make in response to certain stimuli, such as positive suggestion.

In time, new discoveries led to changes in therapeutic approach. As they were found effective, they were passed on to future generations as part of oral tradition and later written. In the 3,500-year-old Egyptian papyri and the 3,000-year-old Babylonian cuneiform tablets, we find evidence that a multitude of different natural products were mixed into pumice or potion to treat illnesses. In general, the role ascribed to these medicinals was to drive out the "demons" that had invaded the bodies. In the tradition of their predecessors, healers believed, by and large, that it was still the "soul" of an herb that appeased the "soul" of an offended spirit. In one ancient account, a physician-priest directed his colleagues to combine a medicinal herb, which assuaged the soul, with some bitter substance, generally a form of animal dung, to drive evil spirits away. Such inventive potions served to reinforce the overriding faith in verbal appeals directed to spirits. Even today, while modern medicine no longer attributes disease to evil spirits, people still accept bitterness in certain preparations, believing in its enhanced ability to cure. Perhaps the sense of sacrifice or pain must accompany the treatment in order for the medicine to work.

The earliest written documents, from the 16th to 17th centuries B.C., present details of pathology and diseases, as well as of treatments. In one Egyptian papyrus, discovered by George Ebers in 1872–73, we find complete descriptions of medications used in 1552 B.C., a time when Moses was only 21 years old. They probably represent medicinal preparations that had been passed down to subsequent generations for a thousand or more years. These prescriptions were apparently prepared by an ancestral precursor to our modern pharmacist. The preparations, while hardly like any we use today, represented remedies that had been found to abate disease symptoms. They included whole parts of plants and animals, living and dead. Generally, a special chant accompanied the medication. Verbal appeal was an important component of the therapy.

For diarrhea, the ancient Egyptians suggested a mixture of figs, grapes, sycamore fruit, gum, and yellow ochre—along with a special chant. For headache, "skull of silicrus fish is boiled with oil and the head is rubbed therewith for four days."[1]

The cuneiform tablet writings of ancient Assyria, dating from over 2,500 years ago, also document the mixture of healing substances:[2]

- For a headache, the following direction was given. "Thou shalt beat up fennel in cow's milk or cow's urine, wash his head (therewith), reduce *barhus*, bray (it) press it on his head, annoint with oil . . . "
- For an eye problem this advice was given. "Thou shalt disembowel a yellow frog, mix its gall in curd, apply to the eyes."
- For toothache, people were advised, "Thou shalt slit a leek, rub on the root of the tooth and he shall recover."

These writings highlight the extent of medicinals known and used and the importance placed on their proper preparations and applications.

The prescription of medicinals to the afflicted was not uniformly accepted. As Greek mythology relates, Aesculapius angered the gods by taking the ability to cure disease away from them and giving it to mankind. Aesculapius, regarded by most as an ancient physician and by some as a deity, reportedly made house calls to visit his patients in bed. From writings of this time, we can deduce that he probably used emetics and purgatives, incisions, and ointments. When his medicines failed, he relied on his faith in music and incantations to heal. His disciples, advocates of medicines, were seen as enemies of the traditional priesthood, which believed its members had exclusive power over disease. According to them, offerings should be made not to the patient but to the holy shrines. The Aesculapians, however, who were priests as well as physicians, developed their own religious following and temples. Their delivery of medicinals directly to the ill person clearly defined the movement away from purely spiritual appeal to tangible cures, residing in organic materials found in natural sources.

During a large part of our later recorded history, sickness was attributed to having too much or too little of necessary bodily substances. Ancient Greeks defined illness as the imbalance of four body humors—blood, phlegm, yellow bile, and black bile—that embodied a mixture of four universal qualities: moist, dry, cold, and warm. Hippocrates, and later Aristotle in the 4th century B.C., articulated this fundamental concept in their teachings. In disease, something either had to be replaced or had to be removed in order to restore health. Influenced by this interpretation, medical practitioners often removed humors; hence, the practice of using leeches attached to the body to suck blood. Under the guidance of this theory, physicians tested and found other effective natural substances. We know today that these substances, such as plant leaves and roots, contained active chemical ingredients, including antibiotics, that were the agents responsible for the relief of symptoms and cure of the disease. The treatments became classified according to their abilities to correct disturbances in the body, such as fever, rapid heart beat, and muscle weakness.

These ideas formed the rationale for a more organized approach to disease, introduced in the second century by a Greek physician named Galen (130–200 A.D.), who is perhaps history's most influential doctor (Figure 3.1). His more than 22 volumes of teachings greatly influenced medicine and attracted followers for more than 14 centuries. It was Galen who first showed that blood, not air, flowed through arteries. He also proved that urine came from the kidneys. But his fame came from his approach to healing, which led to the discovery and use of other substances as medicinals. Galen based his medical theories and ideas on how natural products found in their native surroundings fit the particular needs of the

Figure 3.1. Claude Galen (130–200 A.D.) prepared and used natural substances as medicinals based on their presumed ability to correct an imbalance in the body's humors. Galen chose substances that were opposite in quality to the bodily humor that he believed was out of balance. His influence on medical therapeutics lasted more than one thousand years. (Rare books section, Countway Medical Library, Boston.)

body as defined by the "humors." Believing "contraria contrarius curantum," or "that which is opposite cures," he was led to try interesting, new substances. Galen chose an item because it appeared to represent one of the four universal qualities making up the human temperament and gave it to patients based on its ability to restore what he considered absent or off balance. For instance, vinegar was recommended for the burning heart. He borrowed from the old Greek writings, widely from Hippocrates, and added much more of his own scholarship. Some estimate that he more than doubled the medical literature of the time.

The "galenicals" he gathered were simple organic or mineral ingredients. No substance was outside the realm of potential use—the bark of trees, the juices of berries, or algae found in still waters. Galen's preparations were, by their very essence, hard to standardize but were more understandable and more directed to particular disease symptoms than those prominent in the years preceding him. Some were prepared by Galen and his followers and given to the patient; others were made by the patients themselves on advice of the Galenist physicians. No details on amounts were provided. Galen let each patient or physician decide. By consequence, during this extended period of Galen's influence, drug-making by pharmaceutical professionals, who were beginning to surface, progressed very slowly.

Although viewed as separate entities, medicine (the science of diagnosis and treatment) and pharmacy (the science of drug production and drug activity) evolved alongside each other. Certain early physicians devoted their energies to both. Aristotle carried his own medicines with him and had them available to give directly to his patients. To a large extent, so did Galen and his followers. But the pharmacist emerged where his expertise was needed, particularly with the demand for defined medicinal substances. In the 13th and 14th centuries in England and Germany, apothecary shops appeared and a real separation of physician and pharmacist took place. With the establishment of the pharmacist and the apothecary, attention was increasingly focused on the disease and its symptoms.

Consumer confidence and quality control of the product became important early on. In the 13th century, Frederick II, emperor of Spain and Italy, issued an edict that required every medical man to give information against any pharmacist who sold "bad" medicine:

Every physician given a license to practice must take an oath that he shall faithfully fulfill all the requirements of the law, and in addition, whenever it comes to his knowledge that any apothecary has for sale drugs that are of less than normal strength, he shall report him to the court. . . .[3]

He went on to disallow any physician from owning an apothecary himself, a desirable mandate not practiced in parts of the world today. The Emperor saw clearly how a conflict of interest could emerge.

Today we obtain our medications from pharmacies, generally through the prescription of a physician. The pharmacy represents, therefore, the physical provider of medication and also assures its quality. The two professionals, doctor and pharmacist, are thus intertwined in the delivery of medicine to the patient. In certain countries and for certain drugs, however, medicines can be obtained without a doctor's prescription, that is, as an over-the-counter item. This practice, which we shall discuss further, has broken the tie between these two professions, permitting and encouraging self-medication.

Galen's influence extended into the 16th century. Then Paracelsus, the son of a country physician from Basel, introduced methods for extracting the active components. Not readily accepted by his peers because of his flamboyant style and ideas, he argued for understanding the essence of medical treatment. He simplified and gave uniformity to Galen's prescriptions. But he took a vastly different approach from the established Galenical method. He treated the diseased organ, not the symptom. He discarded the concept of the "humors." In fact, he publicly burned the works of Galen.

In contrast to Galen, who chose medicinals that represented the opposite of the disease symptoms, Paracelsus believed in the doctrine of "signatures" or "similars." Thus, the flower or the leaf of a plant that most closely resembled the diseased or-

gan was often selected to heal the organ. Historians tell us that
the discovery of digitalis, the single most important drug used
to treat heart disease today, came from the ancient, traditional
use of the extract of the heart-shaped foxglove leaf to treat
symptoms then that we now know were related to the heart.

Instead of Galen's ill-defined proportions, Paracelsus and
followers described exact amounts of particular ingredients to
be used. More than ever before, the pharmacy began to find
its role in society. This novel approach, however, was not accepted universally, and, throughout the 17th century, followers of Paracelsus remained in conflict with the Galenists.

The therapeutics of the Middle Ages and Renaissance continued to be a mixture of superstition from ancient times and
experimental daring of the great physicians of the day. Potions, strange mixtures concocted for good and evil intent and
used throughout recorded ancient civilization, continued in
use into the Middle Ages. As Shakespeare reminded us in the
witches' song in his play *Macbeth* (Act IV, Scene 1):

> *Fillet of a fenny snake*
> *In the caldron boil and bake*
> *Eye of newt and toe of frog*
> *Wool of bat and tongue of dog*
> *Adders' fork and blindworm's sting*
> *Lizard's leg and howlet's wing*
> *For a charm of powerful trouble*
> *Like a Hell broth boil and bubble.*

Belief that disease is caused by evil spirits held sway. Into
the 18th century, people wore purple amulets around their
necks to ward off the plague and other diseases. They contained bits of frog, other animals, and the ever-potent animal
dung. Often extracts of human skulls taken from dead bodies
were part of these preparations. Exorcisms, used to drive out

altered disease states in the human body, continued into the late 1800s.

But the times were being primed for the appearance of "modern" medicines, that is, those bottled and sold as preparations to relieve health problems. Throughout the 17th and 18th centuries, various medicines became commonly available for a variety of ailments. Some from England were imported to the United States. Advertisements for these medications filled almanacs in the United States and England. As early as 1685, Samuel Atkins carried this advertisement in his first almanac:

> Some experienced medicines, sold by William Bradford at Philadelphia. Charles Marshall's Spiritus Mundus, being an excellent medicine against all sorts of Fevers and Agues, Surfeits, Gripes, Pleurisies, etc. A present remedy for the Gravel and Stone, which seldom fails to give ease in half an hour.[4]

The practice continued into the 18th century. Nathaniel Whittimore from Boston offered in 1721, "Sundry very excellent medicines found out to cure both hot and cold gouts, dropsies, consumptions, perilous coughs, fevers, ague and most other diseases incident to Mankind ... To be had at a reasonable price, of N. Whittemore."

These advertisements for over-the-counter medications epitomize the already prevalent trend toward self-treatment. This was further realized in whole books devoted to self-medication. To some extent these books fulfilled a real need; they also played on people's search for easy cures. One book by John Theobald first appeared in 1764 and was already in a third edition by the end of the same year (Figure 3.2, next page). In it, Theobald put together a compendium of remedies that he had collected from different sources. He explained that "these receipts are published chiefly for the use of persons residing

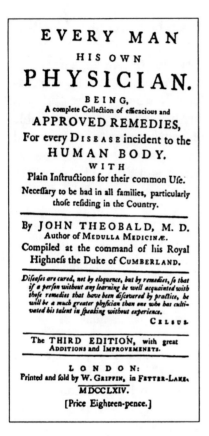

EVERY MAN

HIS OWN

PHYSICIAN.

BEING,

A complete Collection of efficacious and

APPROVED REMEDIES,

For every DISEASE incident to the

HUMAN BODY.

WITH

Plain Instructions for their common Use.

Necessary to be had in all families, particularly
those residing in the Country.

By JOHN THEOBALD, M. D.

Author of MEDULLA MEDICINÆ.

Compiled at the command of his Royal
Highness the Duke of CUMBERLAND.

*Diseases are cured, not by eloquence, but by remedies, so that
if a person without any learning be well acquainted with
those remedies that have been discovered by practice, he
will be a much greater physician than one who has culti-
vated his talent in speaking without experience.*

CELSUS.

The THIRD EDITION, with great
ADDITIONS and IMPROVEMENTS.

LONDON:

Printed and sold by W. GRIFFIN, in FETTER-LANE.

MDCCLXIV.

[Price Eighteen-pence.]

*Figure 3.2.   Almanacs of this
kind were popular in the 17th
century and into the 18th century.
Many books published in England
were sold in the United States.
These books formalized "home
remedies" and propagated self-
medication (Rare books section,
Countway Medical Library,
Boston).*

in the country whose convenience or abilities will not allow of the attendance of a physician or apothecary."[5]

The ingredients of these remedies were in part galenicals but had the details of a modern pharmaceutical preparation. For instance, one such home remedy for pleurisy states, "Bleed frequently till the pain abates, apply a blister to the side, and take half a pint of the following infusion twice a day: take fresh horsedung six ounces and pour on it a pint of boiling Pennyroyal water, strain it when cold and add a quarter of an ounce of Venice treacle, mix for use." Theobold credited this remedy to

Figure 3.3. *Louis Pasteur (1822–1895), the French chemist responsible for successfully arguing the "germ theory of disease," revolutionized our view of infectious diseases and of the approach to therapy (Rare books section, Countway Medical Library, Boston).*

the London physician John Quincy, who published a list of dispensaries during the early part of the 18th century.

It can be argued that these books and almanacs may have offered benefits to some, in terms of easy harmless "home remedies," but they opened up opportunities for quackery, playing on people's wishes to find a ready cure for their ailments. Most pertinent to present-day antibiotic misuse, however, was the encouragement for self-medication. This practice, prominent today, has potentially harmful effects not only on the individual but, in the case of antibiotics, on the sustained efficacy of these drugs. While present-day societies have reaped the rewards of past discovery, they have also inherited a potentially harmful relaxed attitude toward medications, particularly evident in regard to antibiotics.

A significant development in understanding disease appeared in the 19th century and led to yet another change in the direction of drug discovery. Although the concept of a diseased state of man, rather than a causal agent, was still in vogue, as we noted earlier, Louis Pasteur, working and writing in Paris at the time, produced convincing observations that "êtres vivants," "living creatures" or microorganisms, were causing human disease (Figure 3.3). Linking these microscopic beings to disease was a major step into the modern era of medicine. With the "germ" as a causative agent, the scene was set for tremendous advancement in the field of medical science.

This framework encouraged scientists to look for drugs as defined therapeutic entities directed to fight bacteria. The ability of these agents to kill bacteria and cure previously fatal diseases was nothing less than a miracle. Their discovery satisfied the never-ending appeal of miraculous curing agents able to restore well-being to the patient and to society.

The mindset of the individuals looking for new drugs and the attitude of the public toward medicines have shaped historical developments of medicine and in turn, antibiotics. Self-medication and the ready availability of medical products has played into the present-day attitude that antibiotics are cure-alls. A naive confidence that antibiotic use is only beneficial has led to misuse and overuse and the consequent selection of mutant forms of bacteria resistant to antibiotics' killing effects.

chapter four

Antibiotic Resistance

Microbial Adaptation and Evolution

Today most infectious-disease causing bacteria that were previously universally susceptible to antibiotics are resistant to at least some antibiotics and, in many instances, to a large number of drugs. We must face this unsettling situation now, only 100 years since the recognition that bacteria cause disease and only 60 years since the discovery of antibiotics.

When antibiotics came into being, they were a godsend. Natural substances made by one microorganism could inhibit growth and kill another. Scientists learned to produce, harvest, and purify these substances for treatment of diseases caused by microorganisms. The dramatic effect of antibiotics in curing previously fatal diseases led to enormous expectations. Even minor symptoms, once left to our own body defenses, were given over to drug therapy, in many cases to these new "miracle" agents. But there was an unexpected consequence to this reliance on antibiotics. Bacteria developed ways to resist them. With increased and prolonged use came selection of bacteria that were no longer killed by the antibiotic. These strains prop-

agated and took their places in the environment, coming back
to cause infections that were not cured by these drugs.

How did bacteria "learn" to withstand the onslaught of antibiotics? The answer has revealed an unexpected panoply of
genes and transferable genetic elements that exist in bacteria
and endow their bacterial hosts with the ability to resist these
curing agents.

Bacterial Plasmids

Bacteria, like all living beings, must be able to cope with and
even adapt to changing environments in order to survive. The
traits encoded by genes in the DNA of their single chromosome are often not enough to ensure their survival in the face
of adverse conditions. Therefore, bacteria, through evolution,
have acquired and maintained supplemental genetic information in the form of accessory pieces of DNA that are separate
from the chromosome itself. These so-called "plasmids" exist
as independent, self-duplicating genetic elements—like
minichromosomes—carrying as few as three and as many as
300 different additional genes. Anywhere from one to as
many as a thousand copies of a plasmid may exist in a cell.
Many different plasmids can reside in the same cell. The information that the plasmids carry enables bacteria to perform
new functions and engender new products that are not part of
their chromosomal genetic repertoires (Figure 4.1).

The traits borne by plasmids are numerous and versatile.
They enable bacteria to adhere to the cells lining the human
gastrointestinal tract so that these bacteria can withstand the
continuous flow of food residues passing through it. They help
their host bacterium survive a sudden change in the environment, such as extremes of temperature. Unlike the physical and
physiological changes that occur in trees and plants with sea-
sons, or that occur in animals that hibernate during winter,
these plasmid-borne "survival" traits are there to be called into

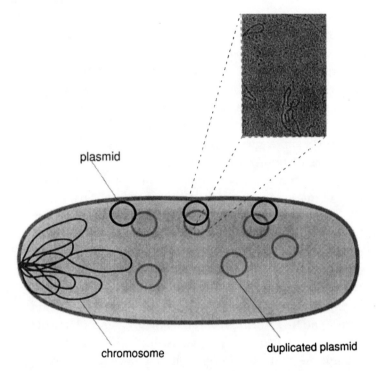

plasmid

chromosome

duplicated plasmid

Figure 4.1 *Plasmids are small, circular pieces of self-replicating, double-stranded DNA that are accessory genetic elements in the cell. There may be as few as one or as many as a thousand copies in a cell. They provide other traits not specified by the cell's single chromosome. The inset is an electron micrograph of a plasmid (18,480-fold magnification) isolated from* Escherichia coli *(Bonnie Marshall, Tufts University School of Medicine). (Figure not drawn to scale.)*

play at any time. Thus, bacteria bearing accessory traits can better accommodate the sludge of sewage systems, the fast moving waters of rivers and streams, the rise and fall of temperatures, the killing effects of ultraviolet light from the sun, and the changing humidity of soils. But perhaps the most important function of plasmids in the bacteria that we confront today is their ability to help their bacterial hosts thwart the action of antibiotics. Not all plasmids bear all the characteristics discussed above, including the genes for antibiotic resistance, but the numbers that do bear resistance traits are increasing, so that few if any disease-causing bacteria lack antibiotic resistance genes.

Plasmids, like bacterial viruses, multiply within bacteria. They are visible only by the electron microscope, being more than a million-fold smaller than bacteria (Figure 4.1). Unlike viruses, plasmids lack a protective outer protein coat and, therefore, cannot survive outside the bacterial cell. They have no chance of multiplying except in the cell and are thus dependent on the cell. In one sense, although they are not independent microorganisms, they exist as a kind of parasite of the cell. Their very presence illustrates the evolution of a mutually helpful relationship between these genetic elements and bacteria. Since their destiny rests entirely with the host bacterium, they cannot afford to kill this host. Thus, viruses and plasmids are guided by a different rationale in their continued existence. The plasmid, like the faithful servant, depends on its host and, in return, protects the life of its host by providing needed survival traits. The virus, like a Trojan horse, gets through the host wall barrier and, once inside, goes on to kill the host cell when multiplying its progeny. A virus can afford to be more selfish than a plasmid since it can survive as an entity apart from the cell; however, it too must get into a cell in order to make copies of itself.

One poignant example of how bacteria and plasmids can form interdependent relationships comes from an experiment performed by Richard Lenski and his associates at Michigan State University. They introduced a plasmid into a bacterial cell and noticed that it was only temporarily accepted before being lost. Since the plasmid carried a trait providing resistance to the antibiotic chloramphenicol, Lenski added chloramphenicol to the culture of the bacteria. Under the protection of the plasmid-mediated chloramphenicol resistance, the bacteria grew through many generations, after which they removed the drug and looked at growth. To the delight of the investigators, the plasmid now stayed stably in the growing bacterium. In other words, the host bacterium had made an accommodation for the plasmid. The investigators then tried to rid the host bacterium of its plasmid. To their surprise, the growth of the bacterial cell was affected—growth appeared dependent on the plasmid. This was a clear example of evolution. Initially the plasmid needed the cell in order to reproduce, but the cell rejected the plasmid until it supplied a mechanism that protected the cell from the antibiotic. Later, the roles reversed—now the cell had need of the plasmid, not just for its protection against the antibiotic but for its own growth.[1]

Plasmids are not static elements. They are constantly subject to change by either losing or acquiring new genes. Two plasmids in the same bacterial cell can combine to form one large plasmid or to exchange pieces of their DNA. Often these exchanges involve genes for antibiotic resistance. Thus, a single bacterium can acquire multiple antibiotic resistance genes on its favorite plasmid. By exchanging and picking up different genes, one extrachromosomal element can emerge with the ability to provide its host with traits for wide environmental survival, not only new ways to get nutrients, but also new ways to prevent being killed.

Emergence of Resistance Plasmids

Soon after the introduction of penicillin into clinical medicine, bacteria insensitive to the antibiotic appeared. At first, and for many years afterward, these penicillin-resistant bacteria were found in the hospitals where most of the penicillin was being used. Resistant hospital strains were different from the mutant strains that scientists had already isolated in the laboratory. Whereas the laboratory bacterial mutants were resistant to relatively small amounts of penicillin presumably by being less permeable to the drug, the resistant strains that emerged in hospital patients were resistant to large concentrations of the drug. The reason was that hospital strains had acquired a plasmid that enabled the cell to destroy penicillin. Increasing the quantity of penicillin did not help because these resistant bacteria were able to destroy large amounts of the antibiotic. These unexpected findings produced a sobering effect on the optimism that followed the discovery of penicillin. They showed that bacteria had developed a means to protect themselves in a totally unforeseen way. Plasmids, whose existence was virtually unknown until resistance was uncovered, posed quite a threat to the therapeutic miracles that penicillin had brought. Once their presence was noted, their impact on public health soon became realized as patients failed to get better despite penicillin therapy.

Discovery of Transferable Resistance

Our knowledge of the existence of transferable antibiotic resistance plasmids is relatively new and came more than ten years after the discovery of pencillin-resistant staphylococci. In 1959, a bacterial dysentery plaguing numbers of patients in Japan was linked to the bacterium *Shigella dysenteriae*. What was unique about this bacterium was not the disease it caused, but its ability to resist four different kinds of antibacterial agents available at that time, namely, tetracycline, sulfonamide, streptomycin, and chloramphenicol. Multiple-drug resistance had been almost unheard of at the time. Of interest, however, in 1955 before this epidemic, a *S. dysenteriae* with similar resistances was isolated from a Japanese woman on her return from Hong Kong. Since no one else was involved, little was made of the observation at the time.

The 1959 event held more surprises. *Escherichia coli*, normal intestinal bacteria found in the same diarrhea specimens, were also found to be resistant to the *same* four drugs. Not only had scientists discovered a combination of multiple antibiotic resistances not previously seen, but for the first time it was appearing in two different kinds of bacteria simultaneously and in the same place. This was an alarming revelation and the Japanese scientists knew it.

Let us return to penicillin resistance. When it appeared in bacteria, the resistance gene specified the production of an enzyme that destroyed penicillin. This resistance enzyme affected only penicillin; it did not touch sulfonamides, the only other antibacterial agents then in use. Based on what was known about mutants at the time, this resistance could have been the result of a mutation on the bacterial chromosome. Later it was shown to reside on a plasmid. In the case of these multiresistant *Shigella*, it was difficult to even imagine single mutations as the basis for resistance to four different drugs. Each mutation occurs rarely, only once in every 10 million to 100 million multiplications of bacteria. By extrapolating from standard mutation rates, Japanese scientists realized that the resistance to four different kinds of antibiotics in a single microorganism would have required a seemingly unattainable frequency of chromosome mutations. Even if each mutation occurred once in 10 million, mutations to four drugs would have needed 10 million × 10 million × 10 million × 10 million or 10^{28} doublings! This realization led the astute Japanese workers to look for a different genetic basis for multiple drug resistance. They guessed that the resistance traits might be associated with genes *not* on the chromosome. Evidence for "extrachromosomal" genes had emerged a decade before when Joshua Lederberg and Edward Tatum, working together, described sexual exchange in *E. coli*. Traits in one bacterium could be transferred to another if the two had contact. Later the phenomenon was linked to the transfer of extrachromosomal sex factors, called fertility or "F" factors. They and others soon reported that bacteria bearing these F factors could exchange genes on their chromosomes. Occasionally some of the chromosomal genes remained associated with the F factors.

The finding of the same four resistances in two different kinds of bacteria from the same diarrhea specimen provided the impetus for scientists to look for an F factor–like transfer. It did indeed exist. Like F factors, the transferable elements were also plasmids. They were called "R" (resistance) factors to distinguish them from F factors. Unlike F factors, whose transfer was limited to a very small group of related bacteria, multiple resistance was transferable among a wide number of bacterial types. Furthermore, it was revealed that R factors carried genes and traits not normally found on the chromosome, that is, they came from other bacterial hosts.

The discovery of R factors was both exciting and worrisome. Their existence implied that resistances could be carried in the relatively harmless gut bacterium *E. coli* and could be transferred to other bacterial species harmful to man, such as the *Shigella dysenteriae* that caused dysentery in the Japanese patients. In one area, 60% of *Shigella* isolated were resistant, of which no fewer than 90% were multidrug-resistant. Another bacterial family that could accept these plasmids was the *Salmonellae*, whose members cause diarrhea, blood and bone infections, and typhoid fever.

Soon after, reports of transferable plasmids bearing multiple drug resistance came from England, Germany, the United States, and elsewhere. By 1966, more than half of about 300 *E. coli* strains from feces and urine of patients at the Pretoria Hospital in South Africa showed resistance to one or more of the antibacterial drugs. At the same time, almost 25% of *Salmonella* strains isolated in a Boston hospital were multidrug-resistant and carried R factors. This phenomenon was not occurring just in Japan—it was happening worldwide.

The discovery of transferable R factors, forty years ago, opened the eyes of microbiologists and medical scientists to a breadth of gene spread never before imagined. Transfer of resistance genes could occur among bacterial species more genetically and evolutionarily distant than a horse is from a cow.

Though not fully realized at the time, these findings predicted the widespread nature of antibiotic resistance we face today.

Origins of Resistance Genes:
Impact of Antibiotics

Genes for resistance are not new creations. We now know that they appeared, albeit in low frequency, in environmental bacterial species long before they entered bacteria that cause human diseases. Many kinds of bacteria carry resistance plasmids, which very likely protect them from the killing effects of antibiotics and other naturally occurring substances. After all, penicillin and other antibiotics are produced in nature by microorganisms. Some data suggest that resistance genes evolved from genes found in the very microorganisms that produce antibiotics—the soil bacteria. This would be a likely place for them to reside in order to protect these antibiotic producers from their own killing products. We can speculate that resistance genes somehow escaped from soil microorganisms and, after passage and evolution in other bacteria, have entered those that have direct contact with humans.

A number of studies revealed that resistance genes existed before the development and clinical use of antibiotics. In a mid-1960s study of the feces from 47 Kalahari bushmen who had no known contact with other people or with antibiotics, as well as fecal samples from over 300 wild animals in South Africa and Rhodesia (now Zimbabwe), low but detectable numbers of resistant bacteria were found. None of the resistances were transferable. Other studies in "antibiotic-virgin" areas also showed resistant genes in bacteria and these transferred to other bacteria.

One 1969 study examined the frequency of R factors in the intestinal flora of people living in the bush of the Solomon Islands, where antibiotics had not been introduced. Soil bacteria were also studied. Among 40 isolates, two—one from soil and one an *E. coli* from a native living there—contained resistant bacteria bearing transferable R factors. At about the same time, studies in a community in north Borneo, where antibiotics had not been used, also revealed the presence of antibiotic-resistant *E. coli* bearing transferable resistance. In all studies, although they were not common, resistant bacteria delivered a clear message—the resistance genes were *not* newly created by the use of antibiotics. They were already present where antibiotics had never been introduced.

While human usage of antibiotics did not somehow *create* antibiotic resistance genes, it certainly has contributed to the increase in their numbers and the numbers of resistant bacteria. By introducing large quantities of these drugs into the environment, we have drastically altered the ecology of microbes. We have unwittingly given a selective advantage to resistant bacteria.

Today, everywhere, we see the consequences of the widespread massive use of antibiotics. With antibiotics on their side, resistant strains have emerged "victorious" in the world of microbial competition. In certain parts of the world, antibiotic-resistant strains of common bacteria have edged out those susceptible to antibiotics. But the advantage given to resistant bacteria is evident only if an antibiotic is present. Otherwise, resistant and susceptible bacteria are indistinguishable by size, color, growth, and reproductive ability. The prior existence of resistance genes in nature explains why they could appear relatively soon after antibiotics became therapeutic agents. The finding illustrates how nature continues to move toward a balance by imbuing the wily bacteria with the means to survive and persist despite people's persistent attempts to destroy them.

Antibiotic usage has stimulated evolutionary changes that are unparalleled in recorded biological history. Prior records and studies of bacteria did not suggest they were undergoing evolution more quickly than were other living beings. But artificial selection by man-made drugs has fostered changes that are moving at an extremely rapid pace. During almost six decades of antibiotic use, common bacteria appeared with combinations of genes coding for resistance to multiple antibiotics; some are resistant to more than ten *different* drugs. Strains of five different disease-causing bacteria exist today that are resistant to all drugs we have in our medical armamentarium. We shall discuss them later. Suffice it to say that they can be acquired in communities as well as in hospitals. For certain resistant bacteria, like the pneumococci and the staphylococci, we may be forced into "the antibiotic of last resort" for serious infections. The multidrug resistance phenomenon has occurred through the joining together of different and even rarely found resistance genes onto common plasmids. Geneticists, fascinated by their appearances, and clinicians awed by their consequences, are moved to try to understand just how these genetic elements were created and maintained.

Origin of Plasmids

The discovery of plasmids as the genetic vehicles of resistance genes raised questions about their origins. Were plasmids a recent creation, like a new disease, or did they exist before, perhaps in a different environment?

Naomi Datta and colleagues at the Royal Postgraduate Medical School in London examined over 300 different clinical specimens of *E. coli* and other intestinal bacteria that had been isolated from humans and stored during the period 1917 to 1954. Most of the specimens predated any major clinical use of antibiotics. None of the isolated specimens bore a transferable resistance. The only resistance found was in a microorganism naturally resistant to tetracycline. More importantly, the scientists showed that this strain collection contained plasmids—the same kinds of plasmids we see today—only *none bore antibiotic resistance genes*. This finding concurred with the examination of fecal samples from the Kalahari bushmen and animals in South

Africa, where larger numbers of bacteria still showed low frequency of resistant bacteria.

An investigation from our laboratory in Boston in the early 1980s addressed this same question about plasmid origins in another natural environment. We examined the levels of resistance in the gut bacteria of nonhuman primates, namely, baboons living without human contact in the wild savannah of Amboseli National Park in Kenya. Our on-site investigator, Rosalind Rolland, a second-year Tufts University veterinary student, flew to Kenya with boxes of disposable plates, pipettes, flasks, and powdered nutrients—all the supplies required for the three-month field project. Before 4 o'clock each morning, she crawled out of her tent into the Land Rover. She and a team of Cornell anthropologists led by Glenn Hausfater drove 40 kilometers into the wild brush of the national reserve (Figure 4.2). Feces from about 50 baboons were collected and studied soon after they were excreted. The behavioral sociologists knew each animal by name and family ties, so each fecal sample could be assigned to a particular baboon. In this way, single samples from each baboon were examined and members of the same baboon family were compared. The investigators found only low levels of resistant bacteria in the fecal samples. Some of the resistances were on transferable plasmids. Of interest, the few resistant strains identified appeared in the intestinal flora of members of the same baboon family.

These and other studies substantiate that resistance genes are not new, nor are plasmids. They have been around for a long time.

Gene Exchange: Conjugation, Transposition, Transduction, and Transformation

The process by which bacteria share genetic material is as intricate and surprising as the fact that it occurs at all. In one

Figure 4.2. *Baboons* (Papio cynocephalus) *in their natural habitat in a national park in Kenya. The fecal flora from these wild animals had little, if any, antibiotic resistance.*

kind of bacterial mating called "conjugation," a fascinating but not fully understood event occurs. First, the bacterial cell bearing the plasmid produces a fine filamentous protein structure called a "pilus," which reaches out to another bacterium. Upon contact, the pilus draws the two bacteria together. Then the "donor" bacterium makes a duplicate of its plasmid and passes its copy (there can be more than one) to the other cell. Both cells now carry the same resistance plasmid (Figure 4.3, next page). The event can occur in minutes and causes the creation of both a new resistant strain and a new donor. As transfers continue, new and old donors find new recipients and an exponential increase in resistant strains occurs. The transfer process requires such specialized mating apparati, consisting of ten to fifteen different proteins, that scientists believe these proteins have evolved solely for the purpose of the genetic exchanges. Gene transfer must be integral and critical to the overall survival of bacteria, providing a way for

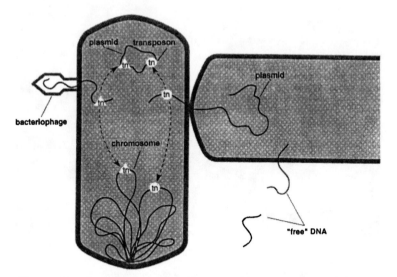

Figure 4.3. *Conjugation via plasmids, transposition via transposons (tn), transformation by naked, "free" DNA and transduction via phages are common means by which genetic material flows from one bacterial cell to another. Transfer of genes takes place among bacteria of all types (Bonnie Marshall, Tufts University School of Medicine).*

them to adapt to difficult conditions. It is a means of producing great diversity and enormous genetic flexibility in the face of changing environmental threats. One survivor can produce new copies of itself, as well as recruit new resistant neighbors.

There is even more complexity and breadth to gene exchange. Small plasmids, which cannot direct their own transfer, enter into a new bacterium by "riding on the backs" of larger plasmids. As before, it is the duplicate plasmid that moves. Ensuing events can further favor the spread of the plasmid copies or its genes. For example, if the new host contains a resident plasmid that can transfer itself, these small plasmids can use it to move into yet other kinds of bacteria. Once in these new hosts, plasmids can spread further. Plasmids entering new types of bacteria can move with their new hosts to environments not visited before. So we see the same kinds of plasmids in bacteria inhabiting the intestinal tracts of humans, as well as those of animals, and in bacteria that live on other surfaces of the body. The same plasmids are found in marine bacteria and soil bacteria. Sometimes, however, the plasmid can find a hostile environment within its new host. In this case, it does not get duplicated, and, therefore, is not donated to new progeny. Thus, it is lost when the original host dies.

Perhaps one of the largest geographic spreads of a plasmid was documented by Thomas O'Brien and his associates of the Brigham and Women's Hospital in Boston. They noted a similarity in a multiresistance plasmid from one of their hospital patients and one reported five years earlier from Seattle, Washington. After genetic sleuthing, these investigators showed that this same plasmid, in different bacterial hosts, had made its way into nine different states and even as far as Caracas, Venezuela. This was intercontinental spread on what they called an "epidemic plasmid."

Other bacteria, notably the enterococci, which we mentioned before, have evolved another kind of mating system. These bacteria secrete substances called pheromones, attractants, which cause two different cells, often called "mating types," to clump together. While closely attached, the two bacteria exchange whole plasmids or pieces of them (Figure 4.4, next page). This aggregation presumably causes a fusion of the cell membranes and an unimpeded free exchange of elements inside the cell, including the plasmid bearing its genes. Streptococci and staphylococci also produce sex pheromones that attract other bacteria of the same or even different types. The resemblance of this microbial mating system to that of other life forms is remarkable. Living creatures as diverse as insects, goldfish, and birds reportedly attract opposite mating

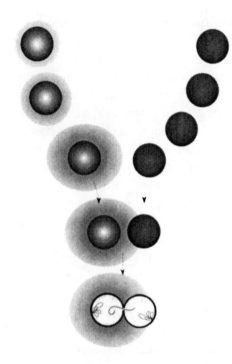

Figure 4.4. *Pheromone-induced genetic exchange among enterococci is another way by which plasmids and genes are exchanged. The donor (left) produces a substance, a pheromone, that draws another bacterium (right) to it. Once together, a genetic exchange takes place. This form of transfer appears in other gram-positive bacteria as well, such as* Staphylococcus *(Bonnie Marshall, Tufts University School of Medicine).*

types by producing pheromones. Even men and women release pheromones, body scents, that attract the opposite sex.

Resistance transfer may occur in other ways. We are learning that bacteria exchange genes without the need for their plasmids to remain in the new cell. This is possible because the resistance gene (or genes) resides on yet smaller pieces of DNA, called "transposons," which can jump from one piece of DNA, such as a plasmid, or chromosome to another and vice versa (see Figure 4.3).

Transposons would do well on a Darwinian scale—they have strong survival potential. Unlike plasmids, they do not rely on a particular host cell or any particular host DNA molecule in order to exist or multiply. Transposons easily become part of diverse microbial species because they "jump ship" onto the host chromosome or onto a resident plasmid already stably docked in the cell. For instance, a plasmid can enter *E. coli* from *Hemophilus influenzae* and deliver its resistance gene, but cannot survive itself. It does not find a place to hitch up. The transposon has another option. It can jump onto the new host chromosome or onto a resident plasmid. While the new host may lose the plasmid and even its copy, the transposon with its resistance information will remain with the new cell since it has found a stable place in the new host. In an analogous way, the common pneumococcus, which causes lobar pneumonia, exchanges resistance genes that are on its chromosome with other streptococci. They do so by moving transposons, called "conjugal transposons," into the new cell.

A relatively new kind of transposon was discovered through the pioneering work of Ruth Hall in Australia.[2] Called an "integron," this genetic element acts like a Venus's-flytrap by attracting resistance genes to it and then capturing them one by one into a single site in the chromosome or a plasmid. The integron, found in many different types of bacteria, has helped to explain the emergence of multidrug resistance, which characterized the 1990s and continues into the present.

Another way that bacteria can transfer genes, both from plasmids and from their chromosomes, is via bacterial viruses, called bacteriophages. Phages, as they are more commonly known, infect only those bacterial hosts that have a particular membrane site to which they can attach. Once there, the phage injects its DNA into the cell. The transferred DNA has two choices: it can multiply rapidly and kill the cell; or it can find a place to sit on the chromosome. If it chooses the chromosome, it may carry pieces of the host chromosome with it when it later pops out of the chromosome to make its progeny. Thus, when the phage multiplies, the chromosomal piece does also and follows the fate of the phage. Upon entering a second host, the phage delivers itself as well as this "carried-along" piece of DNA from its previous host. Gene exchange takes place when the phage and its chromosomal DNA piece integrate into the second host's chromosome. Another way that a phage can transfer genes is via transposons. If the phage has picked up a transposon, it will deliver the transposon to the new host when it injects its DNA. Afterward, the transposon can follow the same route as the phage, or, as it does with plasmids, the transposon can jump off the phage and place itself into a resident plasmid or onto the chromosome of the new host bacterial cell.

Gene transfer can also occur via naked DNA itself. The process, called transformation, involves the pickup by a recipient bacterium of pieces of free DNA released by another bacterium. Once taken up, the DNA can become part of the DNA of the recipient cell.

Transformation is the mechanism principally responsible for the emergence of penicillin-resistant pneumococci. These bacteria acquired pieces of DNA bearing the genes coding for the targets of penicillin, the so-called penicillin binding proteins (PBPs), from harmless other streptococci in the throat. The mosaic PBPs are insensitive to penicillin.

Thus, through many different, but often integrative, transfer processes, pieces of DNA, genes, can move from one bacterial cell to another, including bacteria of very diverse types.

Gene Exchanges In Nature

We now know that bacteria exchange genes readily in nature. Antibiotic resistance has allowed us to see just how extensive these transfers can be, because resistance genes are so easy to identify and follow. By plating on an agar plate containing an antibiotic, investigators can identify strains that are resistant to that drug. By placing antibiotic-impregnated discs on a plate spread with the strain and incubated, scientists can learn how many resistances are present in the strain. More recently, with the advent of gene cloning, each resistance gene can be identified as a special gene, not just as a resistance trait. This can be done by a number of methods. One, called DNA:DNA hybridization, uses a biochemically or radioactively marked strand of DNA of the gene being followed to find its copy, a second strand, on a filter paper bearing DNA from the resistant strains of interest. If a match is there, the marked strand will join to the DNA on the paper. A "hybridization" occurs, which can be noted by the radioactive or biochemical signal. In this way, the exact gene can be tracked among different strains resistant to the same drug.

Another method uses an enzyme that can seek out and find the sought-after gene in an extremely small amount of bacterial DNA. Known as the polymerase chain reaction (PCR), it repeatedly synthesizes the portion of the gene asked for by moving back and forth like an old dot printer to build up more and more copies of the gene. The presence of the gene can then be easily seen in the amplified segment of the DNA by putting the whole reaction mixture on a gelatin-based separation system and staining for DNA.

The hybridization and PCR methods have shown that antibiotic resistance genes, formerly found among a narrow group of bacteria, are present in different kinds of bacteria residing in very different places. It appears that previously susceptible bacterial types have "picked up" the resistance genes during some kind of contact with resistant bacteria. Resistance genes initially identified in gram-positive bacteria were found in gram-negative bacteria. These kinds of bacteria had not previously been known to exchange genetic material.

For instance, one type of gene, *tet*(M), which specifies tetracycline resistance (there are more than two dozen different types of tetracycline resistance traits), was initially found in enterococci, intestinal bacteria of humans and other animals. The gene was soon recognized in other very different bacterial species that cause diseases of the respiratory and urinary tracts. Marilyn Roberts and her group at the University of Washington have tracked this resistance gene to bacteria frequenting different ecological niches and bearing very different cell wall structures. She recently detected it in the *Mycobacterium* family of bacteria (of which the bacterium causing tuberculosis is a member) and in the *Treponema* bacteria found in the mouth. Of concern, if gene transfer occurs to *Treponema pallidum*, the cause of syphilis, it would limit the use of tetracycline, a drug of second choice after penicillin, for treatment of this sexually transmitted disease.

Let's imagine that different bacteria find themselves confronted by an area saturated with tetracycline. In order to enter and survive, they must become resistant to the drug. The survivors are those that received the resistance gene from a donor before going in. The others die or escape elsewhere (Figure 4.5). Today, *tet*(M) has been picked up by pathogens and nonpathogens alike, all resistant to tetracyclines. Many nonpathogens living in the urogenital or respiratory tracts bear the gene. Although they are no trouble to us, they become reservoirs of the gene and potential "donors" to new pathogens entering the scene. The microbial reservoirs include both aerobic and anaerobic bacteria, many of which were never before known to exchange genes. The *tet*(M) example has revolutionized our view of "wide" when we speak of wide microbial spread of resistance genes.

Staphylococci with the penicillinase gene were first detected over 50 years ago—having appeared during the first uses of penicillin. Until recently, the gene seemed confined to this type of bacteria. Then, Barbara Murray and colleagues in Texas found that enterococci, intestinal bacteria that we have discussed before, began to break down penicillins for the first time. In fact, this ability further thwarted antibiotic treatment. Surprisingly, after DNA:DNA hybridizations were performed, they found that the new gene in the enterococcus was

Figure 4.5. *Tetracycline resistance specified by the* tet(M) *resistance determinant is common in bacteria associated with humans, especially in bacteria in the respiratory and urogenital tracts. The high frequency of the gene suggests that donors are plentiful and recipients are all too eager to obtain this lifesaving resistance determinant (Herbert Hächler, University of Zurich, Zurich, Switzerland).*

not original—it was the old gene from staphylococcus, having found its way into a new host. It took almost 50 years for this apparent transfer to take place. The gene is not an exact copy but has some subtle changes that may have made it acceptable in the enterococcus. The penicillinase gene is present on multiresistance plasmids that are transferable among other enterococci. Such an event is troubling since such a transferable gene would certainly wreak medical havoc if passed to the Group A streptococci, a group of gram-positive bacteria that causes "strep throat" and "scarlet fever." So far, these bacteria are extremely unusual among gram-positive cocci in that they are still sensitive to penicillins.

Some form of transposonlike transfer is the possible route of entry of the staphylococcal penicillinase gene into enterococci. Such is also the presumed route by which the ampicillin resistance gene came into *Hemophilus influenzae*. This gene, first noted in the 1960s, was later shown to reside on a transposon on plasmids in *Escherichia coli* and other gut bacteria. Not until the mid-1970s was the same resistance gene and part of the transposon found unexpectedly on plasmids in resistant strains of *H. influenzae*. The plasmids in *Hemophilus* were not those found in *E. coli*—only the resistance transposon was the same. A similar process begins to explain how the same ampicillin resistance transposon appeared in the very different bacterial species, *Neisseria gonorrhoeae*, that causes the venereal disease gonorrhea. It made *Neisseria* resistant to penicillin. Once again, the resistance gene was the same as that initially found in *E. coli*, only now it was on a plasmid found commonly in *Neisseria*. Since there are common plasmids found in *N. gonorrhoeae* and *H. influenzae*, we cannot be sure whether the transposon jumped onto the plasmid in *Neisseria* and then went to *Hemophilus* or vice versa. Alternatively, it could have happened independently in both species. Scientists are still trying to discover the actual pathway of this exchange. What is clear, however, is that such diverse exchanges can and do take place.

Today, we know that genes bearing different traits, originally considered confined to certain bacterial types that share similarity of shape or cell wall, are now found among bacteria of very different sizes, shapes, and colors. These include rodlike and spherelike bacteria and those that grow with or without air. While these exchanges may be rare events, there do not appear to be conditions that prohibit such exchanges from occurring if potential donors and recipients are given appropriate circumstances for such an exchange. This seeming dissolution of boundaries between categories of bacteria has completely changed scientists' views of microbiology. One begins to see bacteria not as individual species but as a vast array of interacting constituents of an integrated microbial world (Figure 4.6, next page).

Nontransferable Resistances: Still A Problem

Resistance may spread even if it is not on a transferable element. Strains of bacteria resistant to the relatively new fluoroquinolone group of antimicrobials such as norfloxacin, ofloxacin, levofloxacin, and ciprofloxacin have steadily increased over the past decade. These drugs are used for a number of infections, including urinary tract, intestinal, and bone infections. Resistance, when it appears, is mediated by spontaneous mutations in genes naturally present on the cell's chromosome that code for the target of the quinolones. The bacteria with the mutant genes now express a protein product insensitive to the antibiotic. Despite the presence of the fluoroquinolone, these resistant forms survive and propagate.

Fortunately, so far, none of the fluoroquinolone resistance traits have emerged on transferable elements. Therefore, for the moment the resistance problem lies with the host bacterium and efforts can be directed at it, with less concern about spread of the gene to neighboring bacteria. While this latter feature may offer some confinement of the resistance trait, we are learning that the new resistant hosts themselves are sufficiently mobile that they are spreading globally and at an increasing frequency. Most notable are the multiresistant *Staphylococcus aureus* strains, which have added chromosomal fluoroquinolone resistance to their plasmid, transposon, and other resistance genes. *E. coli* and *Pseudomonas* are also appearing with fluoroquinolone resistance at unexpectedly high frequencies.

Rifampin resistance also results from a mutation in a gene on the bacterial chromosome. This drug is used for ear infections, resistant skin infections, and tuberculosis. Today, a major problem in the treatment of tuberculosis is the appearance

Figure 4.6. *Bacteria are not single populations, but part of a vast interactive microbial world exchanging plasmids and genes, allowing adaptation to changing environments (Bonnie Marshall, Tufts University School of Medicine).*

of a resistant tubercle bacillus that does not respond to rifampin, isoniazid, or other agents previously successful in curing this disease. And these mutants confront public health officials in countries worldwide. Thus, while these resistances are not on transferable elements, their appearance in this disease-causing bacterium has created a major deterrent to cure and a major world health problem. We shall discuss later the devastating impact of these multidrug-resistant bacteria in New York City and in many parts of the world.

Methicillin, as we discussed earlier, was synthesized to treat staphylococci that produced the penicillin-degrading enzyme ß-lactamase. Being insensitive to the enzyme, methicillin seemed a clear winner. But to everyone's dismay, methicillin-resistant mutants appeared, first in northern Europe and then worldwide. Again, this resistance gene resides on the cell chromosome, making its host cell wall insensitive to the drug and rendering methicillin useless against the infectious disease caused by the bacteria.

Another chromosomally located resistance determinant is one that specifies destruction of cephalosporin-type antibiotics. These cephalosporinase genes are located on the chromosomes of certain gram-negative bacteria. Generally, these enzymes are produced in very small amounts and so the microorganisms appear to be sensitive to the cephalosporins. Once treatment with one of these cephalosporins begins, however, a small but significant fraction of cells shows an increase in production of the inactivating enzyme. By this means, the microorganism becomes fully resistant. The increasing use of the newer, so-called "third-generation" cephalosporins, together with this potential resistance gene, has caused *Enterobacter* to become the third leading cause of hospital infections caused by gram-negative bacteria today.

In one study involving multiple medical centers that looked at the kinds of bacteria isolated from the bloodstreams of hospital patients, those patients receiving a third-generation cephalosporin were three times more likely to have multidrug-resistant *Enterobacter* as the causative agent than those who did not receive the cephalosporin. Moreover, those patients in whom *Enterobacter* were found had a twofold higher chance of dying from the disease than those who had an antibiotic-susceptible one. Thus, by an uncommon chromosomal trait, an uncommon pathogen has become very prominent in hospital infections. The study's authors suggest that "more judicious use of third-generation cephalosporins" may decrease the incidence of these hospital infections and also the mortality from them.

Vancomycin Resistance in *Staphylococcus aureus*

When this book was first published, one of the disaster scenarios imagined involved a multidrug-resistant *Staphylococcus aureus* that was no longer susceptible to vancomycin. This event has occurred.

The first reported strain of a vancomycin-insensitive, methicillin-resistant *Staphylococcus aureus* appeared in Japan in 1996. A four-month-old boy developed an infection at the site of recent thoracic surgery. Although he received treatment with vancomycin for almost a month, the infection persisted. Only with the addition of several other antibiotics, one of which was new in Japan, was the infection cured. The Japanese clinicians had never faced such a formidable foe as this MRSA, which showed an unusually low level of susceptibility to vancomycin and to multiple other antibiotics. This event was only the beginning. Within a year, other vancomycin-insensitive strains appeared in Japan, the U.S., and elsewhere, most recently in Korea. At least two patients have died because of vancomycin failure. Interestingly, the *S. aureus*, instead of picking up the vancomycin resistance transposon from the enterococcus, which had already emerged with it, became resistant on its own through mutations on its chromosome. The cell wall was now insensitive to the action of vancomycin.

Diverse Mechanisms for Resistance

Bacteria have acquired fascinating and novel ways to survive antibiotics. Some do not let the antibiotic in or export it out; others chemically modify the antibiotic so it is no longer active; others simply destroy it; and still others replace a sensitive antibiotic target with one that is insensitive to the drug.

Decreased Drug Entry

In order for antibiotics to work, they must penetrate the cell. Many do so by making use of transport systems already in the bacteria. Thus, in a suicidal fashion, bacteria furnish special transport systems for some growth-inhibiting substances and supply their own routes for death. For this reason, altered transport into the cell was one of the resistance mechanisms expected in resistant bacteria and was presumably the mechanism for penicillin resistance first seen in the laboratory mutants produced by Alexander Fleming. But resistance by this mechanism is generally not very powerful since the block in uptake is not great and can often be overcome by giving more of the drug. Decreased permeability, however, when accompanying other mechanisms of resistance, can provide the host with very high levels of resistance that are insurmountable by increased antibiotic dosage.

Another more potent way to prevent uptake of an antibiotic into the bacterial cell is to increase its export from the cell. This is how many tetracycline-resistant bacteria survive. By a unique mechanism, the resistant cell pumps tetracycline out of the cell faster than it can accumulate inside (Figure 4.7, next page). This pump is made of a protein produced in the cell by the tetracycline resistance gene. In order to work, it requires energy from the cell. The efflux of tetracycline is very efficient, allowing resistant cells to survive up to 100 times the therapeutic dose of tetracycline. Active efflux as a mechanism for bacterial drug resistance has also been found for other antibiotics, such as erythromycin, chloramphenicol, ciprofloxacin, and other toxic elements, such as heavy metals.

Inactivation of the Antibiotic

In contrast to the way the resistant cell deals with tetracycline, other resistance mechanisms are dependent on specific de-

Figure 4.7.   One mechanism for tetracycline resistance involves actively pumping the drug out of the cell, keeping it away from its active target, the ribosome (Herbert Hächler, University of Zurich, Zurich, Switzerland).

structive or modifying enzymes that defuse the power of the antibiotic. Such enzymes have amazed investigators, not only by their specificity for a particular drug but also by the broad variety of destructive and modifying enzymes that exist for the same antibiotic. Under the direction of the resistance genes, cells destroy penicillins by penicillinases and cephalosporins by cephalosporinases. There are more than 90 different kinds of penicillin/cephalosporin-inactivating enzymes specified by resistance genes. The enzymes can be distinguished by their sizes and by their abilities to inactivate different types of penicillins and cephalosporins.

Enzymes alter, and so inactivate, streptomycin, kanamycin, and other drugs of the structurally related "aminoglycoside" group by placing a chemical residue on the drug. The modified drug has trouble getting into the cell and, therefore, cannot bind to the cell's protein-synthesizing machinery, the ribosomes, where it normally inhibits protein synthesis. Similarly, resistance to chloramphenicol is also mediated by an enzyme that modifies and so destroys the drug's activity.

Alteration in the Antibiotic Target

Instead of acting on the antibiotic itself, other mechanisms affect the target of the antibiotic's action in the bacterium. This is one way that bacteria become resistant to the fluoroquinolones and rifampin, drugs we discussed earlier. By a cell mutation, the enzyme (on which either fluoroquinolones or rifampin acts) changes, making the cell insensitive to that antibiotic.

In a similar fashion, but by a different mechanism, the erythromycin resistance gene, usually carried on plasmids, leads to a change in the ribosome, the site of action of erythromycin. The modification does not affect the ability of this important cellular structure to make proteins, but does eliminate its binding site for the antibiotic. A second kind of mechanism for tetracycline resistance, specified by the tet(M) gene, also works by somehow altering its target, the ribosome. A protein product of this tetracycline resistance gene "protects" the ribosome from the inhibitory action of tetracycline by keeping the drug away from its target (Figure 4.8, next page).

Substitution of Antibiotic-Insensitive Targets

Resistance to trimethoprim and the sulfonamides also involves a mechanism that leaves these synthetic antimicrobials unchanged. Normally, the antimicrobials act by inhibiting key enzymes needed for reproducing the chromosome of the bacterial cell. In resistant bacteria, the drug is not altered, nor is the host bacterium changed. Instead the resistant cell produces a different enzyme, which can substitute for the one on which the antimicrobial acts, only this new one is not inhib-

Figure 4.8. *A second mechanism for tetracycline resistance shields the ribosome from tetracycline, thus preventing the drug from inhibiting protein synthesis (Herbert Hächler, University of Zurich, Zurich, Switzerland).*

ited by the drug. In the presence of trimethoprim-insensitive and sulfonamide-insensitive enzymes, the cell survives contact with these growth-inhibitory drugs.

In view of the discovery that there are naturally occurring resistance genes able to deal with these synthetic antibacterial agents, we must rethink our idea that resistance genes were created and sustained in bacteria in order to protect them from antibiotics. While this may still be true in some cases, quite possibly resistance genes have other purposes and have merely been selected by the antibiotics we use because they "happen" to allow the bacterial host to resist the drug. Once so selected and present in the environment, however, use of these drugs will augment the frequency of resistance genes. And this is exactly what happens.

In one study in the mid-1980s, American students entering Mexico for the first time were placed on the drug combination trimethoprim/sulfamethoxazole as prophylaxis for diarrhea during their two-week stay. This practice is not generally accepted today. In any case, over this time period, the intestinal bacterial flora of students taking the drug were examined and compared with the intestinal bacteria of those who were not. There was a rapid appearance of intestinal *E. coli* bearing transferable resistance to both of the drugs in those students taking the antibiotic combination, but not in the control group not ingesting the drug. While these "new" *E. coli* were no health problem to the students, their appearance illustrated the high frequency of these resistance genes already in the Mexican environment at that time and the selective effect of the drugs being taken for the drug-resistant strains.

In a study completed in 1987, almost 10% of first-year students at a Boston medical school were found to harbor *E. coli* that were resistant to this drug combination at a level of 10% or more of the total *E. coli* in their gastrointestinal tracts. The students had no contact with patients and had not been taking any antibiotics for at least a month.

The trimethoprim/sulfamethoxazole combination was introduced in the 1970s. Studies show that in less than one generation of clinical use of this combination, resistant strains had reached levels easily detected in our resident bacterial flora. Normally such resistant *E. coli* would cause no problem, but they serve as reservoirs of these resistance genes. Sometimes even *E. coli* can give trouble. Two leukemia patients in Los Angeles died from bloodstream infections caused by just such a trimethoprim/sulfamethoxazole–resistant *E. coli* that was, until that time, totally unexpected.

The trimethoprim/sulfamethoxazole combination has long been the recommended drug of choice for the treatment of urinary tract infections, a common ailment among women. Within the last few years however, more than 10% of *E. coli*, the commonest cause of urinary tract infections, are resistant to this drug, thus necessitating the choice of another antibiotic. This kind of change in resistance profile is what is troubling attempts to find inexpensive, orally available, and safe medications for common illnesses.

Resistance Mechanisms and the Environment

Because the actions of resistant bacteria do not destroy the tetracyclines, macrolides, trimethoprim, sulfonamides, or the quinolones, these antibiotics can remain intact in the environment unless destroyed by high temperatures or other physical damage, such as ultraviolet light from the sun. Many of the resistance traits for other antibiotics are also non-destructive. In fact, the majority of resistance mechanisms do not inactivate the drugs. Therefore, as active antibiotics, they continue to kill off susceptible bacteria with which they have contact and select surviving resistant forms. The resistant strains have an advantage and become more numerous. Thus, these kinds of resistance mechanisms, unlike the penicillinases, serve only the bacteria that bear them. On the other hand, if resistant bacteria are using mechanisms that inactivate the antibiotic, such as penicillinases, they will remove the antibiotic from the environment. This effect will remove continued selection of resistant strains and protect sensitive bacteria that happen to be in their vicinity. From the medical standpoint, this can be a problem. For instance, a penicillin-susceptible pathogen may be difficult to eradicate in the throat if a penicillinase-producing strain is also there. The ß-lactamase producer protects the susceptible pathogen by destroying the penicillin.

The persistence of antibiotics in the environment after use in people, animals, and agriculture can influence the reservoirs of bacteria bearing antibiotic resistance genes. Antibiotics are deposited in the environment via human and animal excrement in a "post-treatment" phase, where they can continue to select resistant bacteria (Figure 4.9). This period may

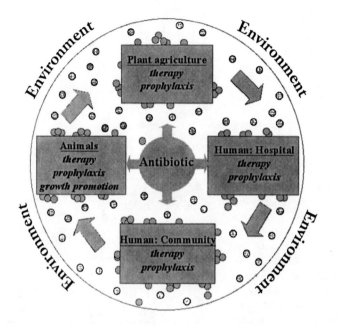

Figure 4.9. *Antibiotics are used in humans, animals, and agriculture for therapy, prophylaxis, and growth promotion. Once provided, antibiotics are discharged into the environment, where they remain active and can continue to select antibiotic-resistant bacteria. (Teresa Barbosa, Tufts University School of Medicine)*

be called their "life after treatment." It is possible that more drug resistance emerges *after*, rather than *during*, treatment (Figure 4.10, next page). After all, therapy is provided at high concentrations of drugs, which would be less likely to select for resistance, while following treatment, the drugs entering the environment are diluted to low levels that enhance selection of resistant microbes. Antibiotics can be recovered from soils plowed with the feces of animals. Antibiotics have been found in municipal waters in Europe and the United States. If the environment sustains this kind of pollution, is it any wonder that resistant strains retain their presence even in locations where the drugs are not being used for therapy?

Figure 4.10. *Given the potentially prolonged period of time during which an antibiotic may remain in the environment after therapeutic use, this presence may be a larger selective force for antibiotic-resistant bacteria than that during treatment. (Teresa Barbosa, Tufts University School of Medicine)*

From the environmental viewpoint, therefore, degradative mechanisms are helpful. They remove the active drug from the environment and so reduce its ability to select for resistant strains. Herein lies another facet of the antibiotic paradox—resistance mechanisms, like the antibiotics themselves, can play both positive (for the environment) and negative (for the patient) roles.

Multiple-Drug Resistance

Single-drug resistance can occur via a chromosomal mutation that generally limits drug entry into the cell or alters the target site of the antibiotic. These kinds of "simple" mutants rarely create a medical problem, since we usually have many alternative active antibiotics from which to choose. Today, we are confounded by the phenomenon of *multiple*-drug resistance and the existence of separate determinants of resistance on plasmids and transposons. Multidrug resistance is the *rule*, not the exception, among resistant bacteria. To some extent, this situation has occurred through the sequential acquisition of each resistance trait following the use of the selecting antibiotic. The first antibiotic began by selecting a single resistance gene. Eventually, however, bacteria resistant to the first antibiotic picked up resistances to others as they were introduced into the environment. The bacteria, however, did not lose the previously acquired resistance traits. It's like a snowball rolling downhill, picking up snow and any debris during its transit, becoming bigger in the process, and not losing what it had acquired before (Figure 4.11, next page). So do plasmids as they "roll" through the environment.

A fascinating correlation was revealed by microbiologist Jacob Kupersztoch of Mexico, who now lives in Texas. He recorded the predominant types of multiresistant *Shigella* present in Mexico and found that they reflected the chronology of different antibiotics being introduced into the country. The most common resistances were to the drugs first introduced in the 1940s, the sulfonamides, followed by those introduced later: penicillin, chloramphenicol, and tetracycline. A similar phenomenon was noted *during* an epidemic of cholera in Tanzania in the mid-1970s. As doctors seized on new drugs, the infecting *Vibrio cholerae* appeared with resistance to each subsequently used antibiotic. Scientists see transposons and integrons as responsible for this process, using plasmids as their vehicles for insertion, duplication, and transfer.

Resistant strains of the gonococcus examined in the U.S. in the past decade showed that tetracycline resistance was often associated with penicillin resistance, a resistance trait that appeared in the organism one or two decades earlier. More striking, those strains resistant to both penicillin and tetracy-

Figure 4.11. *Plasmids pick up resistance genes on transposons as they move through the environment. By retaining previous ones and picking up new ones, they increase in size, like a snowball rolling down a hill (Bonnie Marshall, Tufts University School of Medicine).*

cline had lower susceptibility to two other active drugs, ciprofloxacin and ceftriaxone, than did strains that were penicillin- and tetracycline-susceptible. The prediction was that resistance to the latter two drugs would appear initially among those already resistant to penicillin and tetracycline. In fact, that is what happened in Asia and later in other parts of the world. Gonococci resistant to ciprofloxacin appeared. Today, some strains of this community-acquired infectious disease agent only respond to the cephalosporins, such as ceftriaxone. Given what has happened before, as use of this final drug increases we risk having to confront strains resistant to all four active drugs.

Given enough antibiotic use and its consequent selection of resistant strains, resistance increases and rears a foreboding and Hydralike head. Thus, with time, we see the creation of microorganisms resistant not to just one drug but to multiple drugs. It is the multiply resistant bacteria appearing in different diseases and ecologic settings that truly threaten our ability to treat infections successfully today.

One of the most difficult present-day problems of multidrug resistance faced public health authorities in New York City in the past decade—tuberculosis resistant to multiple drugs. Individuals infected with these resistant bacteria died, despite attempted therapy. The emergence of resistance in the microorganisms is considered the result of patients' not completing a normal course of therapy, inappropriate treatments, and antibiotic misuse. The resistant strains first gained prominence when prison inmates died. The problem was also recognized in intravenous drug users, as well as the indigent and homeless populations. Following the New York City outbreak, two other hospitals in New York State reported the problem. At least eight healthcare workers contracted the disease.

The problem is even worse among immunocompromised patients. For instance, a large proportion of tuberculosis patients nationwide is infected with the AIDS virus, and many now bear resistant strains of TB.

The incidence of tuberculosis began to increase in the United States at the end of the 1970s, even before AIDS appeared on the scene. From this time onward, many TB health programs had their budgets drastically cut or their programs discontinued. The timing of these events was bad. Although resistance was reported periodically, it had never reached dangerous proportions until the 1990s. Drastic measures were needed. Attention was directed both at finding appropriate therapy for the resistant strains and at preventing their spread. Meetings were held in order to alert clinicians and raise awareness of the problem. Suddenly, "TB is out of control in this country," one official remarked at a meeting. Multidrug resistance in this microorganism created truly one of the most critical medical emergencies of the past decade.

Through directly observed therapy (DOT) and public health measures, the New York City health department was able to reduce new cases of resistant TB from 444 in 1992 to 81 in 1996, but at a large cost—over $100 million. Fortunately, the success of this initiative continues today.

Multidrug-resistant (MDR) tuberculosis confronts countries worldwide. The *New York Times* reported MDR TB on all five continents. Among countries in which MDR TB was a major problem were India, Russia, Latvia, Estonia, the Dominican Republic, Argentina, and Ivory Coast. Efforts provided through private foundations and international agencies like WHO and the World Bank are aimed to contain and cure the MDR tuberculosis in these "hot spots" of trouble. The Public Health Research Institute of New York, through funds provided by the Soros Foundation, has focused efforts on the Russian prisons where MDR TB is rampant. They have established diagnostic capabilities, built local infrastructure, and obtained epidemiological data to help change this disastrous situation. Although the U.S. gained control of the problem in the past decade, unless vigilance is continued, these kinds of strains can again become threats in the U.S. as they continue to plague other countries worldwide.

The pneumococcus represents another current, ongoing multidrug resistance problem. In Eastern Europe, Central America, Spain, South Africa, and elsewhere, this microorganism, the cause of infection of one or more of the lobes of the lung, called lobar (pneumococcal) pneumonia, has appeared with resistance to penicillin, erythromycin, and tetracycline as well as trimethoprim/sulfamethoxazole—all first-line drugs for therapy. The result has been a high rate of treatment failures and a search for alternative modes. The choices are slim when the microorganisms are so multiresistant.

Multiple resistance in *Shigella* has been an obstacle to therapy of dysentery in Africa and other developing nations for many years. But the problem has emerged in the United States as well. The Centers for Disease Control and Prevention reported outbreaks of multiply resistant *Shigella* among Native Americans on Hopi and Navajo reservations in Arizona. Of concern was the resistance to trimethoprim, an agent previously effective against multidrug-resistant strains. Farther away, but at about the same time, Bulgaria reported resistance to four to six drugs, including trimethoprim in *Shigella*. And, among over 3,000 isolates of resistant *Shigella* in Vietnam, 90% were insensitive to three or more antibiotics. These findings show the worldwide nature of this multiresistance phenomenon. Without the use of these previously effective drugs, these countries must use more costly newer ones, assuming they are even affordable and available.

Multidrug resistance in *Staphylococcus aureus* ravaged hospital patients in Melbourne, Australia, in the 1980s before public health measures and one antibiotic came to the rescue. We shall discuss this key incident and its ramifications later.

Single Antibiotic Use Leads to Multidrug Resistance

For reasons beyond our present understanding, the continuous use of even a single antibiotic over a period of weeks to months will select bacteria with resistance to different kinds of antibiotics, in addition to the one in use. This multiple resistance is not linked to a single gene or a single mechanism. The phenomenon is again associated with plasmids collecting different transposons. It is easy to understand the selection of multidrug resistance if plasmids already bear more than one resistance determinant. The phenomenon we are addressing, however, is the gradual appearance of more and more resistance in the same bacteria with continued use of the *single* antibiotic. This seeming recruitment of multiple resistance transposons under selection by a single antibiotic is very curious.

Why should bacteria want or need to resist more than the drug with which they are being confronted? The phenomenon has been observed repeatedly. For instance, female patients being treated with only tetracycline for urinary tract infections were found to excrete, in their feces, *E. coli* with increasing numbers of different kinds of resistances as the therapy extended into weeks. The same findings were observed in patients taking tetracycline for treatment of acne. As weeks went by, more and more bacteria in their intestinal tract became resistant to as many as six different antibiotics.

Besides intestinal bacteria, those on the skin have also responded to this chronic use of a single antibiotic. Wesley Kloos from North Carolina State University examined the susceptibility of various types of staphylococci on the skin of patients taking either tetracycline or erythromycin daily for acne. He showed the gradual transition with time from antibiotic susceptible types to those with multiple-drug resistance. Other studies of humans and animals have substantiated the reproducibility of this phenomenon. It usually takes two weeks or more on the antibiotic for the multiresistance to appear. The reason that this recruitment of multiple resistance occurs is still unclear, although the players involved, namely, transposons, integrons, and plasmids, are well known.

Awhile ago, research work in my laboratory revealed this evolution of multidrug resistance even in the absence of plasmids and transposons. While growing a plasmid-free *E. coli* in the isolated environment of a test tube in the presence of small amounts of tetracycline, we obtained bacteria surviving the treatment. Quite unexpectedly, on further study, the same surviving bacteria showed resistance to seven other antibiotics as well. This phenomenon occurred repeatedly with other *E. coli* isolated from feces of different people or from animal feces. Yet these bacteria had no resistance plasmids and no resistance transposons.

With increasing antibiotic contact, the initial mutants emerged with higher and higher levels of resistance. The initial mutation that led to multiresistance has been located in a single site on the *E. coli* chromosome. Many genes on the chromosome are needed to produce all these different resistances, but all are under the control of this single, mutated chromosomal site. Even more surprising, the resistances were not limited to naturally occurring antibiotics, but also to the newer synthetic antimicrobials, the fluoroquinolones, such as norfloxacin and ciprofloxacin. This same multiple resistance locus has been found on the chromosomes of other types of bacteria, thus enlarging the kinds of bacteria potentially subject to this form of mutation.

These environmental and test-tube studies show that bacteria must have some intrinsic, yet unexplained, reason for displaying multiple resistance when confronted with a single drug. It is almost as if bacteria strategically anticipate the confrontation of other drugs when they resist one. If resistance genes are present in the environment, as on transposons and plasmids, the surviving bacteria recruit these genes, thereby acquiring immediate high-level resistance. Otherwise, they still have a chromosomal mutation that provides low-level protection and survival of at least some of the cell population.

Multiresistance:
A General Biological Phenomenon

Multidrug resistance is not unique to bacteria, but occurs in other microorganisms, including insects, infectious parasites, and human cancer cells (Figure 4.12). Agricultural farmers are faced with destructive insects resistant and multiresistant to pesticides. Malaria was initially controlled by attacking the mosquito, carrier of the malarial parasite, with DDT. Today the resurgence of malaria can be explained by the appearance of mosquitos that not only have resistance to DDT, but that carry resistance to other insecticides as well.

In a large part of the world, the malaria parasite itself has become resistant to chloroquine as well as to other drugs used to treat malaria patients. Today, this multidrug resistance has become a leading obstacle to curing the disease and protecting against infection.

Treatment of human cancers with one growth-inhibiting drug can lead to the emergence of small numbers of surviving cells that bear resistance to that drug as well as to other structurally different chemotherapeutic agents. Here, as in the mutated *E. coli* and in the malaria parasite, the trait for these resistances already existed in silent form on the chromosomes of the cell, but mutated to overt expression. Tumors consist of cancer cells with different levels of susceptibility to the anti-cancer drugs. When a patient is treated, those tumor cells with slightly less susceptibility, that is, those that are slightly resistant, become dominant in the tumor because the drugs select and kill off the drug-sensitive tumor cells that compete with the resistant mutants for the blood supply. As with bacterial infections, these resistant cells multiply and become the dominant entity in the tumor. The cancer no longer responds to the therapy. Today, multidrug resistance is a phenomenon that thwarts our ability to cure cancer, perversely mimicking the problem with bacteria.

WINSTON-SALEM JOURNAL

ILLUSTRATION BY JIM STANLEY

Bugs Building Up Immunity to Chemicals

Figure 4.12.   Multidrug resistance is common to bacteria and parasites, linked to overuse of growth-inhibiting agents. This cartoon was inspired by a symposium in Chicago in 1987 at the annual meeting of the American Association for Advancement of Science. Scientists shared data that revealed a resistance problem among different living organisms. (Illustration by Jim Stanley, Winston-Salem Journal, Winston-Salem, North Carolina.)

Bacterial Resistance: A Problem Affecting Decision-Making

Bacterial resistance to antibiotics is not a new creation of the past 50 years. It has, however, become a new clinical problem, because preexistent, naturally occurring plasmids have become equipped with previously rare resistance genes. The combination of resistance genes on transferable plasmids has enhanced the spread of resistance. Bacteria have demonstrated to us a remarkable fluidity in their genetic material.

Under the threat of antibiotics, a small number of them can achieve a tenacious survival mode, either by chromosomal mutation or, more frequently, by acquisition of new genes. These events allow them to persist and grow in the direct path of what had been efficient killing agents, the antibiotics. We now find increased numbers and types of resistant strains, along with new combinations of resistances in even one bacterium. All of this has appeared within the short time span of two generations. We are presently witnessing a massive, unprecedented evolutionary change in bacteria. By developing and using antibiotics, we have, in a sense, caused these events to spiral. We are at a new era of understanding—considerations regarding bacterial resistance must be part of our decision-making and part of our planning for the future of antibiotic therapy. They must include both medical and environmental concerns.

chapter five

The Antibiotic Myth

Antibiotics continue to be our major therapeutic resource for curing and preventing infectious diseases. Their introduction in the 1940s totally revolutionized the treatment of human infections, and the successes of antibiotics continue to prompt their immediate use when an infectious bacterial cause is suspected. The myth of the so-called "miracle drugs" persists today, however, as people unthinkingly demand antibiotics for ailments for which these agents have no value. In turn, their effectiveness is often diminished, tarnishing their reputations and putting us at risk from unresponding infection by drug-resistant forms of bacteria.

Human Use and Abuse

A look at several examples of people and instances where antibiotics have been misused can be illuminating.

Ms. E., an attractive, bright, 25-year-old lawyer fresh from law school, landed a job in one of the well-known 100-member New York City law firms. She had just finished her first set of briefs for one of the senior partners. She was proud of her work and satisfied with her position, but long hours and little sleep had gradually taken their toll. "I must be coming down with a cold," she told the secretary as she walked out wearily that day, suffering from a scratchy throat, achy muscles, and a mild headache. "I hope I'll be in tomorrow, but I'll see." At home she prepared hot soup and tea but relief was only temporary. She had joined a community health plan and decided to make use of it the next day.

"But there's nothing seriously wrong," Dr. R. told her. "It's just a virus. You have no fever. Your throat is red but hardly inflamed. I suggest you get some rest. Take some aspirin. I've taken a throat culture and done a test here in my office. It's negative for the streptococcus that causes 'strep throat.' I seriously doubt that you have anything other than a cold for which you do not need a prescription. The generalized achiness tells me that you've got one of the flu viruses."

"But I need an antibiotic, Doctor," Ms. E. insisted. "I've always gotten an antibiotic before when I've had a cold and it has always helped me."

"Well, that may appear to be the case," replied the doctor. "But if you had symptoms like these, you had a common cold caused by a virus. You would have gotten better without the antibiotic. That's what you have now and antibiotics are not my recommendation."

Ms. E. was not satisfied and, in fact, found herself another physician in the area and got her antibiotic. She changed her health plan. "I can't afford to be sick," she told me. "How do you doctors know that an antibiotic would not help *me*?"

Ms. E., like many young adults, has been brought up on the "antibiotics-work-for-a-cold" myth. In fact, the cold virus is not touched by antibiotics. The French have a wonderful saying that portrays this ineffectiveness: "An untreated cold goes on for seven days; a treated cold lasts a week."

Despite physicians' advice to the contrary, a person searching long enough will eventually find a physician who will prescribe an antibiotic, even when one is not indicated. Success in the search may be influenced by how well the patient knows the physician and the risk that denial of the drug might lead to the physician's losing the patient. To some extent this casual attitude about antibiotics is due to ignorance on both sides, the consumer and the prescriber. The consumer, believing in the miracle drug, knows nothing about the potential harm in taking an antibiotic in a trivial fashion. The physician, worried about losing the patient, may rationalize that a bacterium may be involved but, if pushed, will probably admit that he or she thinks it is likely just a viral cold. Of course, there may also be a tiny minority of physicians who still believe in the powers of antibiotics in all instances.

*   *   *

In another setting, a less subjective factor can influence the patient's ability to obtain the antibiotic. Who is paying for the drug? In the private sector this usually means the patient, and if the patient is willing to buy the medication and the doctor provides the prescription, the antibiotic is obtained. In a prepaid health program, the result may be different. The program foots the bill. The doctors may be less apt to give in to patient demand and patients have less say in the matter. There is no risk to the physician of losing the person as a patient and, in fact, physician prescribing practice is often monitored. Antibiotics and other drugs are generally under closer scrutiny in these instances than in the totally private sector. Although a prepaid program's goal is to provide the best care to the patient, there is a concerted effort to keep costs down. Here there is often an ongoing bureaucratic assessment of the rationale for prescriptions, which does not prevail in the private outpatient arena.

In many parts of the world, such as Mexico, the Caribbean, South America, and Southeast Asia, antibiotics can be obtained directly from physicians or over-the-counter in pharmacies. This setting precludes the need to "plead" or "argue" for the drug. Over-the-counter availability generates and propagates a "laissez-faire" attitude toward medicines that leads to antibiotic misuse. On a visit to Santiago, Chile, to discuss the problem of antibiotic misuse, I stayed at a hotel that happened to be across the street from a pharmacy. Curious, I went over to see how easy it would be to obtain an antibiotic. I did not have to enter the store. In the window were bottles of a number of different antibiotics, all available to the consumer. To my surprise, there was a sale going on. For that week, and only that week, I could get the locally made chloramphenicol for 30% off the list price. If I wanted the American-made product, I could still get a 10% discount (Figure 5.1). While this may seem shocking, it is even more disturbing that a potentially hazardous antibiotic should be dispensed so freely.

In these same countries, only limited supplies of drugs are provided to government clinics for treatment of the vast majority of people living there. When in short supply, antibiotics are prescribed in small amounts so as to reserve them for those in real need. Insufficient supplies dictate shorter periods of treatment and smaller dosages. Herein lies another aspect of the problem. Short courses of therapy, using less of the antibiotic, may not totally cure the disease. In some instances, only the first day's treatment of the antibiotic may be offered to the patient, leaving the rest to be bought at the local pharmacy. This can pose a severe burden to the patient for whom a day's antibiotic can equal a day's pay. Inadequate treatment leads to continued illness and potential spread of the infectious bacteria to other members of the community.

On a more optimistic note, in the year 2000 Chile eliminated over-the-counter sales of antibiotics. This action represents an enormously important public health advance and the

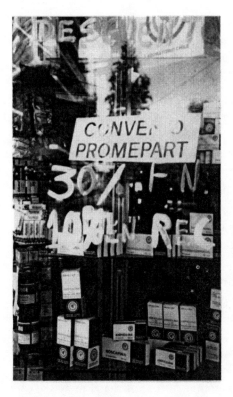

Figure 5.1. *The over-the-counter sale of antibiotics in pharmacies is a common occurrence in Central and South America and other countries of the developing world. During this particular week in Santiago, Chile, there was a sale (DESCUENTO) on chloramphenicol, with 30% off the locally produced product or 10% off the imported product. Other antibiotics were also displayed in the windows and readily available to the consumer.*

first time such a change has been accomplished nationally. Hopefully, it will act as a model for other nations.

*   *   *

While the poor get inadequate amounts of antibiotic, the wealthy in these countries can easily obtain any of these drugs they want. A case in point is Mr. C., a respected 49-year-old businessman from Buenos Aires, who had accumulated millions from his family fortune and from his personal investments. He was the father of five young children and the husband of a lovely 40-year-old woman, a former model in Buenos Aires. An energetic man, he spent more than two-thirds of his day pursuing business ventures but still found time to spend with his family. Mr. C. did not like to be held back by sore throats and mild cold symptoms. While he maintained great faith in the advice and medications given to him by his family physician, he generally treated himself with readily available drugs that he bought at the local pharmacy. On one occasion, however, Mr. C. had had an exceptionally bad cough and fever, on and off for several weeks. He had trouble starting his day because of extreme fatigue. During that time he had been taking several different antibiotics that he had obtained from his pharmacy, to no avail.

Dr. S. noticed an unusual pallor that he had not recognized in Mr. C.'s previous visits over the last ten years. "I think we should get a blood test on you," he said. "I've also noticed some tiny red spots coming up on my legs and arms," Mr. C. added. Dr. S. examined the areas and recognized them as tiny bleeds in the skin. He suspected a serious disease. He looked up and asked, "What kinds of drugs have you gotten your hands on? Did you take any chloramphenicol?" Dr. S. was concerned about a potential critical side effect of this antibiotic—its ability to shut down blood production in the bone marrow and even cause leukemia. "No, not that I'm aware of. I keep a number of these drugs at home, but I don't remember that one," Mr. C. answered.

The blood test on Mr. C. showed him to be anemic, evidenced by a reduction in circulating red cells. His white count was elevated; he had very few platelets, the blood components that help to control bleeding. It was this problem that led to the red marks on his skin. The white cells themselves appeared abnormal. Dr. S. diagnosed acute leukemia.

Mr. C. was flown to a medical center in Boston, where the diagnosis was confirmed. He had a high fever, and his white cell count had climbed to 20 times the normal number and consisted mostly of abnormal-looking white cells. The hematology team put him on a ten-day course of chemotherapeutic drugs and warned that he would become very weak. While the drugs were given to rid his body of all the leukemic cells, each day of therapy brought on worse symptoms. He became nauseated and had to be treated with antinausea drugs. Additionally, he needed antibiotics to treat his infection.

In one arm went the drugs for his leukemia and in the other arm went the high-powered antibiotics for the infection. For some reason, however, the fever did not abate. The intern told Mr. C. that an intestinal bacterium, *Escherichia coli*, was circulating in his bloodstream. What the intern did not share with him was that this particular *E. coli* had proven resistant to *eight* different antibiotics.

Both the intern and the resident had never seen this severe a resistance problem before. A normal *E. coli* should be killed by any of the antibiotics, including ampicillin, tetracycline, cephalosporins, gentamicin, and other members of the aminoglycoside family of antibiotics. Mr. C.'s microorganism was resistant to these and to other penicillins, as well as other highly potent antibiotics. Even the newer members of the cephalosporin family of antibiotics proved ineffective. Later, physicians determined that the resistances were to many of the drugs that Mr. C. had been taking freely over the last ten years. This microorganism had accumulated resistance not only to these but to a vast array of other effective drugs carried on the same plasmid.

Over the ten-day course of chemotherapy, the bone marrow was rid of all detectable leukemic cells. On the 17th day, the bone marrow test showed that Mr. C. had come through the chemotherapy as well as any other patient so treated and should be on his way to an initial remission. But fever and infection persisted. The high doses of antibiotics were not controlling the infection and were troublesome because of their possible interference with the blood's ability to clot. His platelet count was critically low as well. On day 20, with no warning, while speaking to his nurse, his eyes turned upward and he began to shake. He suddenly lost consciousness. When he woke up several hours later he could not talk. He had apparently sustained a bleed in his head. His blood still lacked normal white cells and his body was still ravaged by the multiresistant *E. coli*. Over the next two days, he went further downhill. And on the 22nd day after chemotherapy, with his bone marrow free of detectable leukemia, Mr. C. died of bleeding and overwhelming infection. An autopsy showed that the resistant *E. coli* had produced multiple sites of infection in his liver and other organs.

Although Mr. C.'s leukemia was responding to treatment, his infection was out of control. He succumbed to infection, *not* to leukemia. The cause was a microorganism brought with him into the hospital—one found in his own intestinal tract, the probable result of his own repeated antibiotic usage. Other far-reaching potential consequences of this resistance are troubling and undeniable. Resistant strains selected in one person can move to infect other people. The appearance of this unusual multiply resistant strain of bacteria, "imported" so to speak, could lead to its spread to other hospital patients. Additionally, the genes specifying the multiple resistance could be exchanged among other bacteria native to this new environment. These new recipient bacterial types could associate with other people and even cause disease. Intermittent and repeated antibiotic use, as illustrated in this patient, creates an environment not only of microorganisms resistant to the drug being used but also of bacteria that are resistant to many different antibiotics. As the resistances accumulate, they can be found on one or two plasmids in the bacterial cell. These can be transferred all together to other bacteria. So one new recipient cell can receive the entire resistance "package" of another bacterium. The net result is that many previously powerful, nontoxic, inexpensive, and often lifesaving antibiotics can become useless quickly.

*   *   *

Individual users and physicians frequently abuse antibiotics, but neither is the only culprit. In many instances, it is others making decisions for the individual whom we should fault for their ignorance of the ramifications of such abuse. Under a rationale of prophylaxis, that is, preventive treatment, many well-meaning people are providing antibiotics to tens of thousands of people. Whether it is the mother from a Boston suburb who innocently treats a busload of children with penicillin because one of them has a cold, or a government agency in Indonesia that authorizes giving tetracycline to thousands going on a pilgrimage, the result is the same—killing of sensitive bacteria and recruitment of drug-resistant types.

"One hundred thousand people, pilgrims, are going to Mecca this month," the laboratory technician told me while I was visiting Jakarta, Indonesia. He was referring to a hundred thousand people from all parts of Indonesia who would be traveling by foot, train, and plane. The pilgrimage, a massive trek to Saudi Arabia, was, to many of these people, their life-long dream, and they were determined to make it. The rich and the poor went together. Only their mode of transportation distinguished one from the other.

However, the Indonesian Ministry of Religion, which organized and directed the pilgrimage, was concerned about the possible spread of disease among these people. The most likely devastating disease was cholera. This severe form of diarrhea, caused by the bacterium *Vibrio cholerae*, often spreads among people via contaminated water or food or through close physical contact. For this reason, all foods served on the trains and planes were checked for these disease-causing bacteria, as well as for *Salmonella*, another potential cause of diarrhea. The laboratory I was visiting in 1981 was responsible for these analyses.

Many lives had been lost to infectious diseases during these pilgrimages. So a new approach had been developed whereby each individual was checked for cholera before departure. And then, just in case, each was given the antibiotic tetracycline.

"You mean all 100,000 pilgrims are getting tetracycline?" I asked in a state of disbelief.

"Yes, and for seven days," replied my host. "In fact, the government keeps them in quarantine for this period until they finish taking the drug."

He told me that the Ministry of Religion supplies the antibiotic. It is "dished out of vats like coffee beans." I already knew the answer to my next question but asked anyway. "Is there any control on the quality of the drug?" When antibiotics are given in bulk, it is often necessary to confirm that the drug is fully active. He told me that this was the job of the Food and Drug Administration, but that agency was not involved in the pilgrimage.

This broad-scale use of tetracycline, to "prevent" illness by trying to kill off any infectious bacteria that *might* be there, misses certain key features in the infectious process. First, one microorganism does not cause disease; there must be thousands to millions of them. Second, antibiotics will provide a selective environment for those infectious agents that are resistant to them. Those bacteria that happen to enter our bodies or fall onto our skin take up residence and multiply to dangerously high numbers, all under antibiotic protection. Widespread use of tetracycline has certainly contributed to the increasing number of tetracycline-resistant strains of *V. cholerae* that plague large areas of the developing world. In certain areas, such as parts of Africa, over 50% of the cholera-causing bacteria are now resistant to tetracycline. This antibiotic has always been the drug of choice for treating this disease. Substitute drugs are being tried, but many strains are now becoming resistant to these as well.

Prior to the 1970s, the cholera bacteria were uniformly susceptible to all these drugs. The resistance they have gained had its origins in other kinds of bacteria, such as *E. coli*, that normally live in the gut. By some transfer event, resistances have moved from their previous hosts to new ones, namely, to the *Vibrio cholerae* bacterium.

*   *   *

In the United States, the ease with which an individual can procure antibiotics from physicians and then stockpile them for self-prescription later on is a variation on the same theme we see happening in developing countries. And the numbers of individuals abusing antibiotics here in the United States can be counted in the hundreds of thousands.

Dr. T., an energetic and outgoing psychologist, was tired at the end of her work day, especially after the last, tedious, hour-long session with one of her many clients. She took off to a popular bar near her office in Boston. At age 31 and un-married, she enjoyed chance meetings during these "after-hours" relaxations. On this evening, Mr. S., carrying a draft beer, made his way through the crowd and stopped next to her. "Hi, may I join you?" he asked. Dr. T. was delighted. He looked about her age, maybe a little younger. Their drink to-gether was followed by dinner and then a nightcap at her place. It was not surprising to either of them that they found themselves in bed. Dr. T. was not reluctant, but the fear of unexpected infection could have been a deterrent if it hadn't been for her supply of ampicillin tablets, her choice of antibi-otic protection. She had diligently kept a supply on hand from previous prescriptions for those evenings spent with someone different. She took two pills before and two after. "You never know with whom you might be sleeping!"

This story predates the problem of AIDS, but provides a glimpse of an attitude about antibiotic misuse that persists. It's the self-treatment syndrome combined with the ready avail-ability of antibiotics for self-medication by the individual. Even in the United States this misuse occurs, although there are laws requiring prescriptions to procure these drugs. As far as we know, Dr. T. continues today to use antibiotics on her own, despite our advice to the contrary.

Appropriate use of antibiotics is straightforward and involves the prescription of the drug by a physician to kill off bacteria invading the body of the patient. Clear directives for the use of these drugs come together with the prescription and should be well within the awareness of these educated self-prescribers. But apparently, directives don't provide enough incentive to prompt proper use of antibiotics. Abuse is rampant. This pattern of abuse contributes to the alarming frequency with which resistant bacteria are appearing as causes of disease.

Globally, pneumococci, the cause of ear-infections, pneumonia, and meningitis, have emerged with resistance to penicillin, the drug of first choice, and to other antibiotics as well. These multidrug-resistant, common community-acquired strains thwart treatments, leading to continued illness. In the U.S., penicillin resistance rates have risen from 1–2% in the early 1990s to more than 20% nationwide, with some areas reporting rates of 60% resistance among pneumococcal isolates.

Antibiotics have two major acceptable uses in medicine— treatment and prophylaxis (Figure 5.2). In the area of treatment, antibiotics are given when a known infectious microorganism causes disease. Here the choice can be geared to the microorganism and its expected susceptibility. Another, and perhaps the most common, use is when a bacterial infection is highly suspected by the physician, even though the microorganism has not yet been identified. In this instance, an antibiotic is chosen based on the best clinical judgment. Obviously, it is in this area where there is more room for misuse. Antibiotics are also recommended for disease prophylaxis, that is, to prevent infection at times when there is a known high risk of contracting an infectious illness. Unfortunately, in reality, neither users nor prescribers confine their involvement with antibiotics to only these two conditions.

TREATMENT   **PROPHYLAXIS**

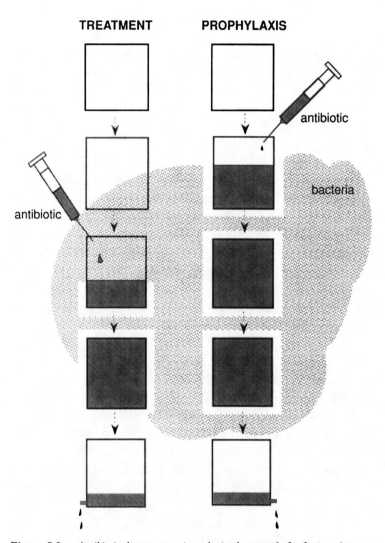

Figure 5.2. Antibiotics have two major roles in the control of infectious diseases: treatment and prophylaxis. The major difference is the timing of the antibiotic. In treatment, the antibiotic is applied after the infection is already present. In prophylaxis, the antibiotic is applied first, preventing infection by invading bacteria such as during certain surgical procedures (Bonnie Marshall, Tufts University School of Medicine).

Selecting an Antibiotic

In the early days of antibiotic discovery, drugs such as penicillin, tetracycline, and streptomycin were developed because of their recognized and unique efficacy against particular disease-causing microorganisms. As more of these antibiotics became available, they were tried on other diseases. Thus the spectrum of bacteria that they killed was established and, in many cases, broadened.

We speak of "broad" and "narrow" spectrum antibiotics in reference to the long or short list of bacterial types affected by the drug. Penicillin, which originally provided a narrow use, has been chemically altered to produce other derivatives that are more broadly effective. Pharmaceutical companies were able to take penicillin's chemical core structure and modify it, thus enlarging its spectrum of activity. Certain penicillin modifications improved the drug's ability to penetrate the outer cell wall of other previously untouchable bacteria. These bacteria included the dreaded *Pseudomonas aeruginosa*, which plagues patients with blood diseases and those undergoing cancer therapy. Practitioners valued the new derivatives for their extended use in killing off yet other kinds of bacteria.

Chemists also modified the core penicillin molecule in order to produce a new kind of penicillin that was not subject to certain resistance mechanisms. The product, methicillin, was not destroyed by enzymes that degraded penicillin in resistant cells. This altered penicillin was able to kill the resistant staphylococcus bacteria that made the penicillin-destroying enzymes.

Today, we have over a hundred antibiotics from which to choose (Table 5.1 pages 130–131). Interestingly, penicillin (and its derivatives), the first antibiotic to be discovered, is still in great use today. This practice reflects, in part, the success of chemical modifications that broaden the activity and counteract resistance. To some extent, the continued use stems from the dilemma of poorer countries where the newer drugs are too expensive to be widely used. Often, the first-line drugs are all that are available, despite their known failure rates against resistant bacteria.

In Bangladesh, for instance, antibiotics are used to treat cholera and shigella dysentery even where the frequency of resistance is at 20%, a level that generally would remove the drug as an option, but there are no other cost-effective drugs available.

The challenge for the physician is to know when and for what kind of bacteria a particular antibiotic should be prescribed. Fever usually indicates invasion of the body by a foreign agent, be it bacterium or virus. It is unusual, for a bacterial infection in the blood, lungs, or other major site in the body not to cause fever, unless the individual's body defenses are subdued by anti-inflammatory drugs that mask fever. Therefore, without fever, antibiotics, as systemic drugs, should be prescribed sparingly. There are, of course, exceptions. Local infections, such as skin abscesses or impetigo, which is a more superficial skin infection, are usually caused by bacteria and should be treated with antibiotics, even though no fever may be present. Sinusitis that lasts more than ten days, especially in children, has a good chance of being bacterial since viral outbreaks usually improve within a week. Fever may not be present. In this instance, antibiotics are recommended because of the high probability of a bacterial cause.

If a bacterial infection is suspected, further diagnostic procedures are generally implemented. A physician will want to identify the specific microorganism before purging the body with large doses of antibiotic. Knowing the kind of bacteria causing the disease helps the physician decide what kind of disease symptoms and signs to expect and what kind of drug to use. Certain bacteria have propensities to infect certain organs, such as the heart, lung, or kidney. Some antibiotics are more effective when given for a bacterial infection of a particular organ because the antibiotic is concentrated in the fluid of that organ, such as the urine in the kidney or the bile in the gallbladder.

Table 5.1.°° Representative antibiotics and antibacterials used in human therapy.

Cephalosporins, 1st generation:	Penicillins/Beta-lactamase inhibitor:	Antituberculosis Agents:
Cefadroxil	Amoxicillin/clavulanate potassium	Ethambutol
Cefazolin	Ampicillin/sulbactam	Cycloserine
Cephalexin	Ticarcillin/clavulanate potassium	Ethionamide
Cephalothin	Piperacillin/tazobactam	Capreomycin
Cephapirin		Isoniazid
Cephradine	**Carbapenems:**	Pyrazinamide
	Meropenem	Rifampin
Cephalosporins, 2nd generation:	Imipenem/cilistatin	Rifapentine
Cefaclor		Rifabutin
Cefamandole	**Monobactams:**	Para-aminosalicylic acid
Cefmetazole	Aztreonam	
Cefonicid		**Sulfonamides:**
Cefotetan	**Aminoglycosides:**	Sulfadiazine
Cefoxitin	Streptomycin	Sulfamethoxazole
Cefprozil	Kanamycin	Sulfisoxazole
Cefuroxime	Amikacin	Sulfamethizole
Loracarbef	Gentamicin	
	Netilmicin	**Oxazolidinones:**
Cephalosporins, 3rd generation:	Tobramycin	Linezolid
Cefdinir	Neomycin	
Cefixime	Paromomycin	**Streptogramins:**
Cefoperazone		Quinupristin/dalfopristin
Cefotaxime	**Macrolides:**	
Ceftazidime	Erythromycin	**Methenamines:**
Ceftibuten	Azithromycin	Methenamine
Ceftizoxime	Clarithromycin	
Ceftriaxone	Dirithromycin	**Nitrofurans:**
Cefpodoxime	Troleandomycin	Nitrofurantoin
		Furazolidone
	Quinolones:	
	Nalidixic acid	
	Oxolinic acid	

Cephalosporins, 4th generation:
Cefepime

Penicillins/Natural:
Penicillin V potassium
Penicillin G aqeous
Penicillin G benzathine
Penicillin G benzathine/procaine

Penicillins/Aminopenicillins:
Amoxicillin
Ampicillin
Bacampicillin

Penicillins/Extended spectrum:
Carbenicillin
Mezlocillin
Piperacillin
Ticarcillin

Penicillins/Penicillinase-resistant:
Cloxacillin
Dicloxacillin
Nafcillin
Oxacillin
Methicillin

Quinolones:
Nalidixic acid
Oxolinic acid

Fluoroquinolones:
Ciprofloxacin
Levofloxacin
Sparfloxacin
Norfloxacin
Gatifloxacin
Gemifloxacin
Ofloxacin
Moxifloxacin
Lomefloxacin
Pefloxacin
Cinoxacin
Trovafloxacin

Tetracyclines:
Tetracycline
Demeclocycline
Doxycycline
Methacycline
Minocycline
Oxytetracycline
Chlortetracycline

Lincosamides:
Lincomycin
Clindamycin

Folate antagonists:
Trimethoprim

Drug combinations:
Trimethoprim/
 sulfamethoxazole
Erythromycin
 ethylsuccinate/
 sulfisoxazole

Other antibiotics:
Chloramphenicol
Vancomycin
Bacitracin
Colistin
Polymyxin B
Spectinomycin
Novobiocin
Metronidazole
Fosfomycin

To secure this information, physicians obtain cultures and perform tests of different areas of the body. In the presence of fever and soreness of the throat or difficulty in swallowing, a physician may want to obtain a swab of the throat and culture it to check for a bacterial culprit, such as streptococcus, which causes "step throat" or scarlet fever (Figure 5.3). If the person has a deep cough, suggestive of a lung infection, one or more samples of the cough secretions, or sputum, are taken and tested for the presence of a known disease-causing bacterium. Initially, a simple test can be done in the office. The sputum sample is smeared on a glass slide that is stained for bacteria, namely, by the Gram stain. The presence of small, round, purple-stained bacteria in chains of two cells, called diplococci, are highly suggestive of pneumococci, which cause so-called "lobar" pneumonia in one or more parts of the lung. With this evidence, and an X-ray confirming pneumonia, the physician would initiate treatment, either at home or in the hospital, depending on the severity of the pneumonia. Definitive identity of the microorganism and an antibiotic susceptibility test would come from culturing the sputum.

If there is burning on urination or pain in the flank areas where the kidneys are located, the physician can usually detect a kidney or bladder infection by direct microscopic viewing of a urine sediment obtained by centrifuging a sample of freshly voided urine. Urine cultures are important in confirming the diagnosis and determining the kind of microorganism involved, including its susceptibility to antibiotics.

Loose or watery bowel movements and cramps lasting a week or more or bloody diarrhea would suggest the need of a stool specimen. These tests tell us about dysenterylike microorganisms, such as *Shigella* or *Campylobacter*, or microorganisms causing milder diarrhea, such as *Vibrio cholerae* and *Salmonella*. Perhaps it is not a bacterial cause at all, but rather a parasite, such as *Giardia*.

A careful examination of the skin, including the perianal

Figure 5.3. The agar plate is an important tool in the work-up of an infectious disease. In this instance, a throat culture is swabbed onto a blood agar plate and the colonies are separated to be visualized and identified. The ß-hemolytic streptococcus, which causes "strep throat," produces a protein that breaks open the animal blood cells suspended in the agar. This is visualized as a halo around the streptococcus colony (arrow).

area, will often tell the observer whether or not there is a deep-seated skin infection that needs to be cultured in order to help decide on a treatment regimen.

If no particular organ or area of the body seems to be the problem and the patient is feverish and appears generally ill, three separate cultures of blood are performed. Since a blood-borne infection would need immediate attention, such patients would usually be transferred to the hospital for these tests and for further evaluation and treatment. The need to check multiple blood samples has come from studies showing that bacteria, even when present, may not be discovered in a single culture at a given point in time.

All clinical specimens go to a bacteriology laboratory where they are put into culture systems that allow growth of any microorganisms present. In the case of blood, bacteriologists inoculate some of the specimen into bottles of growth media, a mixture of salts and nutrients, in order to allow the small numbers of bacteria present to reach detectable levels. Since all internal body samples should be sterile, any growth in the bottles containing blood samples indicates a blood-borne infection. Cultures of urine, feces, and skin all contain normal bacterial inhabitants that must be distinguished from any that could be the cause of the disease. This distinction is made by inoculating the specimens onto a special gelatin medium (like the agar plate first described by Koch in the last century) in round plastic dishes. This plating promotes easy growth of the bacteria into separate colonies and allows identification of the numbers and types of bacteria present in the specimen. In samples from nonsterile sites, the bacteriologist or medical technologist looks discerningly to recognize the harmful bacteria mixed among bacteria normally present in this body material. Certain special tests may be needed to aid in this distinction. For some infections of the bowel or abdomen, bacteria that die in air, the so-called strict anaerobes, may be causing the infection. Therefore, some of the cultures are grown in the presence of nitrogen rather than oxygen.

If the bacteriology laboratory finds disease-causing bacteria in these samples, the microorganism is usually tested for its susceptibility to antibiotics. Before our present-day problem with antibiotic resistance, simple identification of the type of bacteria causing the disease was enough to tell the physician which antibiotic to use. Nowadays we must also determine which antibiotic is likely to be successful.

In many United States hospitals, susceptibility testing is done by an automated machine. Bacteriologists inoculate small amounts of bacteria growing in a medium into separate tubes of a liquid test growth solution, each containing a different antibiotic. If growth occurs in the tube containing an antibiotic, the bacteria are resistant to that antibiotic. Alternatively, some laboratories test by using paper discs (Figure 5.4). The bacteriologist swabs a solution of suspect bacteria onto the surface of an agar plate and lays small paper discs containing antibiotics on top. After a day of incubation at 37°C (98°F), the temperature of the human body, the technologist examines the plates and measures the area around the antibiotic disc where bacteria have not grown. If there is a large area with no lawn of bacteria, the strain is designated susceptible to the antibiotic in that disc.

A

B

Figure 5.4. *Antibiotic testing is done in several different ways; one widely used is the paper disc method. Paper discs impregnated with the antibiotic are placed onto an agar medium already spread with a lawn of the bacteria being tested. During overnight incubation, the antibiotic diffuses into the agar, killing susceptible bacteria. Clear zones around the paper disc indicate bacterial sensitivity to the antibiotic. Growth up to the edge of the disc indicates resistance to the antibiotic. In the cartoon (plate A) the bacteria are resistant to AB-X but susceptible to AB-Y. Plate B contains E. coli from an Indonesian infant with diarrhea. On this plate, the bacteria are susceptible to gentamicin and sulfamethoxazole, moderately susceptible to kanamycin, but resistant to ampicillin, tetracycline, chloramphenicol, and streptomycin. (Cartoon by Herbert Hächler, University of Zurich, Zurich, Switzerland.)*

If there is growth close to the edge of the disc, the strain is resistant. The bacteriology laboratory reports these results to the clinician seeing the patient (Figure 5.5). On the basis of these susceptibility tests, the physician chooses an antibiotic.

The physician must always make a choice of antibiotic based not only on the susceptibility results but also on knowledge of possible allergies of the patient. There is also consideration for the method by which the drug has to be given (orally or parenterally, i.e., by injection into the vein or muscle). Increasingly, although not frequently enough, physicians will also look at the costs of the drugs tested. If two drugs are equally effective, the physician will choose the less expensive. Cost has only recently become a major consideration, in large part because of the high price of some of the newer drugs. For instance, a penicillin treatment typically costs less than a dollar a day, whereas some of the newer antibiotics could cost over one hundred dollars.

In general, use of a single antibiotic is the optimal choice. This avoids problems with side effects, since any one drug can have a side effect and many different side effects could follow use of multiple drugs. Some side effects are expected and occur in most consumers of the antibiotic—these are usually mild and can be tolerated. Others are less common and indicate an allergic reaction—these could be serious. In our population, allergy to drugs is relatively common, second only to hay fever allergy. About 5% of the population may show a reaction to penicillin. While most often this is only a rash, sometimes the reaction can be more severe and the rash may be a warning sign. The antibiotic should be stopped immediately.

The situation can become even more difficult when some penicillin-allergic people show reactions to other drugs with structures related to penicillin. Thus, the physician has to be careful in selecting the alternative drug. If a patient is taking more than one antibiotic and a rash or other adverse reaction develops, it is impossible to know which antibiotic is the cause. Consequently, all drugs must be stopped and a new one

```
CULTURE  WOUND
SOURCE                          RIGHT  FOOT
DATE  FINAL  REPORT             7/08
PRELIM.  ORGANISM  1            MANY  STAPHYLOCOCCUS  SPECIES
FINAL    ORGANISM  1            MANY  STAPHYLOCOCCUS  AUREUS
PRELIM.  ORGANISM  2
FINAL    ORGANISM  2            MODERATE  DIPHTHEROIDS

ORGANISM  NUMBER                       1
AMPICILLIN/SULBACTAM                  >=32  R
CEPHALOTHIN                           >=32  R
CIPROFLOXACIN                          >=4  R
CLINDAMYCIN                            >=8  R
ERYTHROMYCIN                           >=8  R
OXACILLIN                              >=8  R
PENICILLIN                            >=16  R
TRIMETH/SULFA                         <=10  S
VANCOMYCIN                               1  S
MIC  VALUE  IN  MCG/ML
```

Figure 5.5. *An antibiotic susceptibility report on a patient with a bone infection.*
Staphylococcus aureus was isolated and showed multidrug resistance, including
resistance to one of the fluoroquinolones, ciprofloxacin. The microorganism was still
susceptible to the combination of trimethoprim and sulfamethoxazole and to van-
comycin, which, in this case, was the drug of choice.

needs to be started. When several antibiotics are suspected of being the cause of the reaction, the search for an alternative effective drug will be more difficult.

The decision to use an antibiotic is based generally, in the best medical hands, on the benefits compared with the risks associated with its use. In a sick infant suffering from fever and possible dehydration and having little body resilience, the high probability of bacterial infection warrants the use of antibiotics immediately and for the sustained period of the illness. In this case, early use of these drugs can be truly lifesaving. Still, clinicians will take cultures of affected areas—throat, urine, feces—before starting the antibiotic to confirm that the right drug has been started. Sometimes, the initial antibiotic taken may not cure the disease and another will have to be given. However, the microorganisms may have been suppressed in this process. If cultures were not taken prior to starting the first antibiotic, it may be too late at this point to culture and identify the bacteria causing the disease. Thus, there will be no susceptibility test from which to choose an appropriate alternative drug.

In severely ill infants, we are willing to accept possible side effects and biological changes in bacterial flora resulting from antibiotic use because the benefit far exceeds the risk. By a similar reasoning, an elderly, very sick patient with high fever and other signs of obvious infection is presumed to have a bacterial infection. Therefore, after culturing possible sites of infection, antibiotics are begun. The risk of rampant disease in this setting is too great to wait for the culture results. The same decision is not appropriate, however, for an otherwise healthy, young adult who suffers from symptoms attributable to a suspected viral illness. Here, there is time for culturing and waiting the necessary 24 hours for the culture results before beginning an antibiotic. This reasoning is not meant to deny appropriate therapy. It should prevent unnecessary side effects for the individual and remove a purposeless selection of resistant strains for the individual and the community, not to mention saving costs for an already overburdened health care system.

Antibiotics in Disease Prevention

Aside from their use in treating disease, antibiotics have a proper place in preventing threatening bacterial disease. About 30–50% of all antibiotics dispensed in the United States are used for this purpose. The use of penicillin for the victims of the Cocoanut Grove fire in the 1940s was a mixture of therapy and prophylaxis. Some received the drug for infection already present; others were given the antibiotic to prevent infection during skin grafting.

A common prophylactic use of antibiotics is to prevent infection in patients who have had diseases of the valves of their heart or have a heart murmur. The latter indicates some change in the normal functioning of the heart valves that may make them more susceptible to bacterial infections. Damaged valves are at increased risk of infections whenever bacteria circulate in the blood. This situation can occur, for instance, following tooth extractions that might cause transient passage of bacteria from the mouth into the bloodstream. Antibiotics cannot prevent the bacteria from entering the bloodstream, but they can prevent them from "setting up shop." This preventive effect of antibiotics does not need to be prolonged. Therefore, the use is for short periods of time before and immediately after a dental procedure.

Some serious diseases in small children, such as meningitis caused by an invasive type of *Hemophilus* or the meningococcus often suggest the need for prophylactic use of antibiotics in schoolmates as well as household contacts. This practice is done to halt the spread of these life-threatening infections.

Antibiotics are sometimes used to prevent recurrent infections, namely, lobar pneumonia caused by pneumococci, in people who have had their spleens removed for therapy or for rupture after trauma. The spleen produces antibodies that are protective against the bacteria that cause these pneumonias. When the spleen is gone, an antibiotic is often advocated. Today, this practice is being replaced by vaccination against different types of pneumococci and other bacteria before removal of the spleen. Similarly, children who have had rheumatic fever caused by a streptococcus may be maintained for years on penicillin. This practice has been shown to prevent recurrent streptococcus infection, and in particular to protect against serious damage to the heart.

Medical practitioners and surgeons know that antibiotics can be extremely useful in preventing postsurgical infections. These are limited to operations that involve locations and tissues that have a high risk of bacterial contamination, such as operations on the intestinal tract or following trauma with external contaminated objects. For this use, the effectiveness of the antibiotic as a prophylactic agent is, almost by definition, limited to the short period of time before, during, and some-times immediately after surgery. A physician need not prescribe any additional drugs beyond this protective period since the chance of infection from the surgical procedure is over. It is im-portant not to continue these drugs beyond this period unless there is clear evidence of infection. Prolonged use can select for infectious agents circulating in hospitals that are often resistant and emerge in the presence of the antibiotic. Besides the med-ical consequences to the patient, unnecessary antibiotic use is a major contributor to increased hospitalization costs.

Prophylactic use of antibiotics is less rigid in practice since it is based on suspected risk rather than known disease. There-fore, there is room for more error and, in some cases, blatant misuse. In a study of surgery patients in over 50 hospitals in Pennsylvania during the late 1970s, investigators found that, for a large proportion of patients, prophylactic use of antibi-otics for surgery was not limited to the short period before and during surgery but instead was prolonged for the entire hospi-tal stay. This amounted to weeks of antibiotic misuse and long periods of potential selection of antibiotic-resistant strains in these individuals and in the hospital. In cases such as this one, where there was no need for the antibiotic, such continued use tends to lead to the killing off of susceptible, harmless bacteria that normally protect us from invasion by other harmful vari-eties of bacteria. The scenario can be likened to overtreating your lawn with weed killer only to find that the grass is killed off as well; the small number of weeds that survive or enter right after the treatment now have a wide-open area to seed and spread, unimpeded by natural competitors (Figure 5.6).

Fortunately, documentation of this source of misuse and recognition of its harm both biologically and economically has led to vast changes in surgical prophylaxis. Antibiotic prophy-laxis is generally not recommended for "clean" operations ex-cept where the rare chance of infection could produce drastic consequences, such as in heart surgery. For contaminated or po-

Figure 5.6. *Antibiotics kill more than the pathogen to which they are directed. The growth of any other susceptible bacteria will also be inhibited. Once the ecosystem is cleared of bacteria, resistant bacteria can multiply or enter into the noncompetitive arena. The phenomenon can be likened to weeds that have overgrown a lawn where the grass has been completely destroyed by an overdose of herbicides (Bonnie Marshall, Tufts University School of Medicine).*

tentially contaminated procedures, prophylaxis is indicated. Data have fully substantiated the success of the prophylaxis. In a recent study, the timing of antibiotic prophylaxis was found to be crucial—two hours or less before the incision produced the best results. When the antibiotic was given more than two hours before or after the incision, the benefit was less. If the procedure is expected to last for more than four hours, a second dose is recommended, generally within two hours of the first dose. While some believe that no further prophylaxis is required after termination of the operative procedure, others accept a limit of no more than 24 hours following the end of the procedure.

Resistance in the Community: A Consequence of Antibiotic Use and Availability

Urinary tract infections are common, particularly in women. An estimated 40% of the female population will have the problem at least once in their lifetimes. The infecting bacteria usually come from the gut, where they find entry into the bladder through the neighboring urethra. As we discussed earlier, when antibiotics are taken, the susceptible strains of bacteria on human skin, mucous membranes, nasal passages, and in the gastrointestinal tract are killed off by the onslaught of an antibiotic (and in many cases by more than one), leaving room for chance colonization by harmful strains. The longer the use, the greater the effect on our natural flora. Thus, the antibiotic susceptibility of the bowel flora could affect the treatment of a urinary tract infection.

Not all bacteria can cause urinary tract infections. To some extent it is the chance meeting of one type of bacterium with the vulnerable anatomy of a "susceptible" person. There are, for example, some women who will not get an infection even if the potential disease-causing agent is there. In other less usual instances, the infection occurs. The so-called "honeymoon cystitis" is attributed to spread of fecal bacteria to the bladder during periods of frequent sexual activity.

While infections of the bladder are usually easily and successfully treated with antibiotics, some can present real difficulties if the infecting microorganism is resistant. A young woman from Kenya who had had ready access there to all currently available antibiotics came to Boston for consultation because she had a persistent urinary tract infection that did not respond to antibiotics. Once again, the culprit infectious agent was a multiply-resistant common gut bacterium. Only when treated by intravenous therapy with expensive and somewhat toxic drugs, to which she had never been exposed, was she cured of her infection. Time alone will show us for how long.

In some patients, one potential way of treating persistent urinary tract infection is to rid the intestinal tract of the causative bacteria so that the patient will not become reinfected with the same strain. But this poses strategic problems—we cannot sterilize the gut. However, a change of diet might work, since changes in diet, along with bacteria associated normally with the food, can affect the kinds of bacteria that reside in our intestinal tract. In fact, some bacterial strains in our intestinal tract are constantly in flux. If one of these strains is the cause of the urinary tract infection, we can try to get rid of it. To this end, some people suggest eating yogurt. Its efficacy comes from its containing lactobacillus, a common intestinal microorganism that causes us no harm, but colonizes the intestinal tract and, in doing so, can change the flora. Lactobacillus has been advocated and used to help reestablish the normal intestinal flora after antibiotic treatment. We now know that it is not necessarily any type of lactobacillus that can produce this change. Intestinal microbiologists and physicians are presently working on particular strains of lactobacillus that appear to be more effective than others. It may be, as certain animal studies suggest, that lactobacillus can even help rid the intestine of diarrhea-causing *E. coli*, and perhaps other bacteria prone to cause bladder infection.

Lactobacillus forms one of the "core" biologics in the area of "probiotics," a therapeutic option that uses bacteria, bacteriophages, and other non-chemical means to protect against, or alter the course of, infectious organisms. I expect we shall hear more about the use of probiotics in the near future. Already some are commercially available for animals (to prevent salmonella colonization) and for people (to control *Clostridium difficile*-mediated diarrhea and infections by *Pseudomonas aeruginosa*).

A female employee of a Boston hospital had such a persistent urinary tract infection that she was almost constantly on some form of antibiotic treatment. While a cure was usually attained eventually, each treatment required a different antibiotic. Whenever the drugs were stopped, however, the infection resurged. The infection recurred with either the same microorganism or with one showing a new resistance pattern. We advised her to change the place where she normally ate, a local cafeteria, on the chance that her intestinal flora would change, leading to the loss of those microorganisms causing her repeated bladder infections. By coincidence, or by the direct effect of her changing eating establishments, her bladder infections ceased when she stopped eating lunch at this cafeteria. Whether the problem was the bacteria associated with the food she was ingesting or her own intestinal flora that this previous diet encouraged is not clear, but the change in diet appeared to place the bacteria causing her disease at a disadvantage—at least they did not return to bother her. Our interpretation was that she finally eliminated the infecting resistant strains that were constantly recolonizing her gut and causing her urinary tract infections.

A common example of a community-acquired resistant bacterial infection that has emerged under antibiotic selection is the gonococcus bacterium that causes the venereal disease gonorrhea. Previously, penicillin offered an easy cure, but the bacteria have now become resistant to this first-line antibiotic. As noted earlier, this emergence of resistance in a widespread infectious agent in the mid 1970s caused eyebrows to raise and previous doubters to take heed. Antibiotic resistance was not just limited to a few hospital strains or normal intestinal inhabitants. The initial appearance of resistance to penicillin in this microorganism was so new that it allowed the resistant forms to be traced to the brothels of Southeast Asia, one of the aftermaths of the Vietnam War. It was a common practice there for penicillin to be given to women on a regular basis to prevent venereal disease, thereby protecting their serviceman customers. While not proven, the likelihood is that the first resistant gonococcus appeared in Vietnam and was soon transported to Singapore, Europe, and the rest of the world. Today, every country in the world has to deal with this resistant form of a bacterium that was previously susceptible to penicillin.

The rise in penicillin resistance in the gonococcus microorganism necessitated a change to tetracycline, always the second-line agent for patients allergic to penicillin. But today tetracycline has also become ineffective in the face of increasing numbers of tetracycline-resistant gonococcal strains. Their appearance was first documented in New Hampshire in the United States in 1982, but they were discovered soon in other eastern states. Epidemiologists see them spreading worldwide. Isolates have emerged in the Netherlands and other parts of Europe. A sizeable number of the resistant gonococci are multiresistant, that is, resistant to both tetracycline and penicillin. In the last few years, resistance to fluoroquinolones, the next (third) drug of choice for this disease, has joined penicillin and tetracycline resistance among strains of the gonococcus. This situation has caused New York State public health officials and the Centers for Disease Control to recommend using yet another antibiotic, a third generation cephalosporin, as the drug of choice in treating suspected gonorrhea. This is unfortunate since this drug, in contrast to tetracycline, will not simultaneously treat other venereal disease agents that might also be involved. The antibiotic is also more than three times as expensive as tetracycline or penicillin.

Decreased susceptibility to cephalosporins has appeared in certain isolates of this organism. This event prepares us for the possibility that a four-drug-resistant organism will appear. The disease is generally treated with a one-dose regimen observed by the physician in the office or a sexually transmitted disease clinic. When resistance requires more involved treatments or even hospitalizations, we shall see a huge increase in public health dollars, if we can even get the patients to accept this form of treatment. Treating gonorrhea in hospitals will pose a huge obstacle to our ability to cure and control transmission of this community-acquired disease.

Another now-common community resistance problem has developed with *Hemophilus influenzae*, the cause of ear infections in infants, as well as of pneumonia and of meningitis, the infection of the tissue covering the brain. The first appearance of ampicillin-resistant strains was totally unexpected. They were discovered in the early 1970s when two infants in Bethesda, Maryland, failed to respond to ampicillin. They both died before the problem of resistance was diagnosed. The event sparked international concern. But these strains had already begun to appear elsewhere. At the time, Londoners were cautioned about picking up the bacteria from Americans stationed there. In a letter to *Nature* about the potential spread of this resistant *Hemophilus*, the authors warned,

> Since there is considerable intermingling of the American military community with our British hosts, the above data [increased numbers of ampicillin-resistant *Hemophilus* in the UK] suggest the distinct possibility that the American community may act as a source of ampicillin-resistant invasive *H. influenzae* disease for the community at large.[1]

Today, less than twenty years later, ampicillin-resistant and multiresistant *Hemophilus influenzae* is a problem throughout the world. However, a non-drug approach has proven exceedingly successful. A vaccine, prepared against the invasive *H. influenzae* type b strains has effectively reduced *H. influenzae* type b as a cause of upper respiratory tract disease and meningitis.

A more recent example of troubling susceptibility changes involves the group A ß-hemolytic streptococcus. This microorganism causes strep throat, scarlet fever, rheumatic fever, and many other illnesses in children and adults. It was, in fact, the microorganism *Streptococcus pyogenes* that took the life of Jim Henson, the creator of the popular Muppets© of "Sesame Street" fame. Fortunately for us, all group A streptococci are still susceptible to penicillin, the drug of first choice, and treatment is successful when begun soon after infection. However, there has been an alarming increase in resistance of this microorganism to the second drug of choice for treatment—erythromycin.

Erythromycin-resistant group A streptococci were reported more than a decade ago in Japan, and other reports have come out of Canada and Australia. However, they have never reached levels of sustained clinical concern. In Japan, the frequency went down when erythromycin usage was reduced. An important study recently conducted in Finland discovered a dramatic increase in erythromycin-resistant *S. pyogenes* in 1990. The study was initiated two years before, when many erythromycin-resistant isolates from throat swabs were noted in Turku, on the southwestern coast of Finland. The authors established a prospective study to examine whether this was a one-time event or an increasing phenomenon in Finland. The latter concern turned out to be disturbingly true—the problem did not go away and, in fact, was escalating. The investigators made some important observations. There had been more than a threefold increase in the sale of erythromycin in Finland over the previous decade. They also showed that erythromycin-resistant bacteria were the cause of disease in half the patients who did not respond to erythromycin treatment, a finding vastly different from the 96% of patients who carried a susceptible strain and were cured of the disease .

There are several important points that follow from these data. First, a microorganism that causes a common illness worldwide has moved from being highly susceptible to one that is able to resist at least one of the key drugs important in its treatment. For those who are allergic to penicillin, erythromycin is the drug of second choice. Erythromycin is also helpful in the treatment of other disease agents that could complicate upper respiratory tract disease. Secondly, we see that the resistance frequency increased rapidly in this location over the three-year period from 1988 to 1990 and was sustained. There existed also the potential for this resistant microorganism to spread to other parts of the world, as we witnessed with the multidrug-resistant pneumococcus from Spain. Finally, as a consequence of this emergence, more routine antibiotic susceptibility testing was required, particularly for persons allergic to penicillin-like drugs.

At the time, the authors suggested that limiting erythromycin use, as was done in Japan, might help bring the resistance levels down. However, as we noted before, once a resistant strain, (such as an erythromycin-resistant *Streptococcus pyogenes*) emerges in high frequency, it may find its niche alongside the susceptible strains and stay. From there, it can reemerge under erythromycin selection. In fact, Finland initiated a successful public campaign to reduce erythromycin usage. Following a 2-year period of decreased use, resistance rates dropped from almost 20% to less than 10%. Fortunately for Finland, the action was taken soon enough before resistant strains became a stable part of the environment.

Towards the end of the last decade, physicians from the midwestern U.S. described the deaths of children from strains of methicillin-resistant *Staphylococcus aureus* acquired in the community. The organism was different from those found in hospitals. Designated cMRSA, for community-acquired MRSA, these organisms, like those in the hospital, were resistant to methicillin and other penicillins, but unlike hospital isolates, they were not resistant to other antibiotics such as chloramphenicol, tetracycline, and the aminoglycosides. These cMRSA have emerged in the community independent of the hospitals. The key factor is presumably overuse of penicillin-like drugs, but there is also a possible connection with the use of other bacteria-killing agents, namely, the surface antibacterials in household products, as we shall discuss later.

The early recognition of resistance to penicillin in the 1940s heralded a phenomenon now seen commonly with the introduction of each new antibiotic. We practice medicine differently now than in the past. More emphasis than ever is placed on rapid diagnosis and susceptibility testing of the infectious microorganism. While antibiotics are needed and provide immeasurable power to control infectious diseases, their widespread use, often in inappropriate ways and amounts, has contributed to the emergence and rise of resistant bacteria. Given the strong selection of resistant variants by these drugs, the prudent use of antibiotics must become an even greater priority for both the prescriber and the consumer.

chapter six

Antibiotics, Animals, and the Resistance Gene Pool

Of the eight billion animals raised for human consumption in the United States yearly, most receive some antibiotics during their short lifetimes. These include 7.5 billion chickens, about 300 million turkeys, and a million each of cattle and pigs. At any one time, domestic food animals outnumber people in the United States by more than five to one. These figures are important when we assess the effect that antibiotics have on the bacterial flora of these animals that not only share our environment but also end up in our stomachs.

Just as is the case with people, antibiotics are given to domesticated animals for treatment of disease. But quantitatively, much greater amounts of antibiotics are given to animals in small, subtherapeutic levels as a means to improve their growth. When considered in terms of nationwide use, the amount of this subtherapeutic usage is four to five times greater than the amount used for treatment of animal diseases. Antibiotics are also used to treat illnesses in domestic pets, such as dogs and cats, adding another 100–150 million animals to the total number ingesting antibiotics.

In the years following the early success of antibiotics in curing human infections, veterinarians—as well as food producers—looked to these drugs as the answer to infectious disease problems facing livestock. They were not disappointed. The results were so dramatic that antibiotics were soon credited for curing diseases of all kinds, including viral illnesses. This latter claim persists today, even though we now know that antibiotics do not cure viral infections. Most likely, these early observers had treated infections caused by bacteria, not viruses.

In the early 1950s, doses below therapeutic amounts began to be introduced into animal feeds for growth enhancement at about the same time that antibiotics were introduced therapeutically for animals. The discovery of the beneficial effects of small amounts of antibiotics came during the period when food animal producers were searching for "nutritional factors," such as new vitamins, that would improve the growth rates of their animals. Nor was this search limited to animals. There was even a quest to identify factors that would improve the growth of children, particularly in poorer areas of the world where food supplies were limited. A serendipitous discovery propelled the subtherapeutic use of antibiotics as growth promoters into the animal husbandry field.

Robert Stokstad, Thomas Jukes, and colleagues were looking for new microbial sources of "animal protein factor," later found to be vitamin B12, that would improve efficacy of protein utilization and growth in chickens. They were working at Lederle Laboratories, where, in 1947, Benjamin Duggar discovered chlortetracycline, the first member of the tetracycline family of antibiotics. Procuring this drug required harvesting large vats of *Streptomyces aureofaciens*, the soil microorganisms producing the antibiotic. When these investigators tested the microorganism itself, they discovered that it contained a growth enhancer, at first thought to be vitamin B12. But the response was greater than any seen with other vitamin B12 sources. Moreover, when chlortetracycline had been extracted from the microorganisms and the leftover carcasses of the tiny bacterial cells were given to the animals, the growth effect was retained. This meant that the growth-promoting agent was not lost during extraction of the antibiotic. These investigators realized that this material represented an inexpensive source of the "animal protein factor" as well as a growth enhancer for chickens and other animals. Their studies showed that adding even small amounts of the *Streptomyces* mash to chicken feed led to a significant increase in the growth rate of the chickens and weight gain per pound of feed. They initially attributed this effect to a new nutritional "growth factor." They later found that it was nothing other than traces of chlortetracycline remaining in the bacterial carcasses after extraction—in an amount of about 1–5 parts drug per million parts bacterial protein. The potential of such small amounts of antibiotic to improve growth was a powerful discovery that generated a whole new industry. Because of the extremely small amounts of antibiotic, this effect of chlortetracycline was regarded as "nutritional" and not therapeutic by the producers and governmental authorities regulating the food industry. This seemingly innocent interpretation allowed these antibiotics to be sold without prescription. Usually they were added during manufacture of the feed that was then sold at farm dispensaries as a premixed food.

From this time into the 1950s, other antibiotics were tried as growth enhancers by supplementing the animals' feed with small amounts of drugs. Soon penicillin joined chlortetracycline to become one of the two major drugs used as feed additives for cattle, swine, and poultry. Today, many other antibiotics and chemicals have been developed for growth promotion. But penicillins and tetracyclines remain two of the most widely used antibiotics for this purpose in the United States.

Any therapeutic dose may be 10–100 times greater than a dose used in growth promotion. Treatment is directed against a particular infecting microorganism and the goal is to eradicate or control it as quickly as possible. Given the financial constraints of animal husbandry, money is not wasted. The goal is to use these agents for only as long a time as is necessary to rid the animals of infection. Contagious spread of disease can be fast in large herds. This aim is not very different from a doctor's use of antibiotics to treat humans. But herein lies a significant difference between therapeutic and subtherapeutic use. It is not only the quantity but also the total time of usage that is different.

In the case of growth promotion, smaller doses are administered for longer periods of time, for weeks to months. The net result is that as much as 80% of the total amount of antibiotics given yearly to many food animals goes for growth promotion. We are speaking about 15–17 million pounds of antibiotics used subtherapeutically each year in the United States alone. Antibiotics are provided for growth promotion in other countries as well.

Until 1970, growth promotion usage existed in England and other parts of Europe. Then, a committee of British government–appointed microbiologists and physicians investigated the practice and issued a document, The Swann Report, that concluded that this practice was harmful to human health. They showed that subtherapeutic doses for prolonged periods produced a strong selection for resistant bacteria in the animal intestinal flora. They reasoned that these bacteria have a potential risk to people. And there were instances where some bacteria, namely, *Salmonella*, were traced from the animals to disease in people. Since that time, subtherapeutic use of human antimicrobial drugs has been banned in

England, a policy that has been followed in other European countries and Canada as well. Other antibacterial agents, not used in human medicine, are being provided for growth promotion there.

No such legislative ban has been issued in the United States. What is being asked for in the United States is evidence showing a definite link between antibiotic-resistant bacteria that cause human disease and the use of penicillins and tetracyclines for growth promotion in animals. This is not an easy task because these same drugs are used to treat humans and animals; therefore, selection of the resistant bacteria has potentially resulted from either type of usage. New data, however, are coming closer to providing this information. Several studies have traced resistant infections in humans to the same bacteria in animals and animal food products. Subtherapeutic use was implicated in at least one occurrence of resistant infections, specifically in the spread of *Salmonella* from hamburger meat to people living in four western states in the 1980s.

From the data we discussed before, we can estimate that 30 times more animals are being given antibiotics yearly than are humans. Consider with this number the fact that daily animal fecal excretion can be 5–400 times greater than that of humans. For example, the amount of feces excreted by a cow per day is 100 times more than that of a human. If an animal is given an antibiotic, the fecal bacteria that survive the antibiotic treatment are resistant to it. Hence, via their excrement, animals are contributing a large amount of resistant bacteria to the natural environment, much larger amounts than are people. The bacteria in this environment move to new areas and new hosts by many routes, through contact with other animals and insects, as well as with food produce.

Growth promotion enthusiasts in the 1950s asked how these drugs actually caused increased growth. Despite some research into the question, the mechanism of action is still not known today. It may be that even small amounts of antibiotics suppress the growth of certain bacteria that compete for needed nutrients. Or, the antibiotics may eliminate those bacteria that suppress the growth of other intestinal strains that are generating the beneficial nutrients for the animals. Or, the drugs act directly to diminish inflammation in the gastrointestinal tract caused by certain kinds of bacteria. Some still attribute a hidden nutritional value to antibiotics, although no one has shown that the animals can metabolize them for energy. In most instances, the drugs pass through the animals' intestines unchanged. Against a nutritional mechanism of action is the finding that small doses of antibiotics given to laboratory-housed "germ-free" animals do not show a growth promotion effect. These findings strongly imply that bacteria are somehow involved, either as metabolizers (although this is unlikely) or, more likely, as intestinal competitors for nutrients or as causes of inflammation that are suppressed or eliminated by the antibiotic.

Since bacteria must colonize the intestinal tract in order to survive, one plausible explanation is that low levels of antibiotics are inhibiting the production of proteins involved in adhesion and colonization of the intestinal tract. In this way, certain strains that interfere with the animal's ability to gain the full nutritional value of the feed may be eliminated. These bacteria are, therefore, passed out of the intestinal tract with the feces. It is also possible, especially when husbandry sanitation conditions were less stringent than they are today, that these low doses were suppressing disease by inhibiting infecting bacteria during stressful periods. Whatever the reason, and there may be many, for the growth-promotion effect, the intestinal walls of treated animals are thinner than those not treated—more like those observed in germ-free animals.

What was originally viewed as a boon to animal husbandry, and certainly was in its time, has stirred heated controversy in the United States since the 1970s. From the beginning, un-prescribed, over-the-counter use of these valuable agents was frowned upon. It seemed unwise to saturate animals continu-ally with low doses of the same antibiotics needed to treat their diseases. But the initial reports were glowing: animals did not show allergic reactions; people were not knowingly picking up the antibiotic in their food. Surprisingly, resistant strains of bacteria were reportedly not emerging; however, it is apparent that resistance in bacteria was developing from the beginning, but remained undetected. Today, resistance is clearly evident. In fact, wherever food animals are being raised, the bacteria in their intestines and on their skins are largely resistant not to one antibiotic but to many different types of antibiotics.

Notwithstanding the problems caused by the selection of resistant bacteria, the use of antibiotics for growth promotion appears to be having a diminished effect on the animals. More penicillin and tetracycline are now needed to elicit the same increased growth rates they produced in the past. For exam-ple, in the 1950s, 5–10 parts per million of tetracycline were effective; today 50–200 parts per million are needed. The dosage is dependent on the kind of animal and the type of an-tibiotic being used. The trend seems to indicate that growth-promotion doses of these antibiotics are gradually reaching the levels recommended for prevention and therapy. Even with the use of higher amounts of antibiotics, the benefits of growth promotion from this usage are less now than those re-ported thirty years ago. Today, this small growth benefit must be weighed against the environmental and health hazards of a massive selection of resistant bacteria that is a consequence of prolonged antibiotic usage.

Many public interest groups and medical scientists have pe-titioned the U.S. Food and Drug Administration to ban growth-promoting antibiotic usage, notably those involving human therapeutic drugs. Of particular concern are tetracy-clines, which affect a large variety of bacteria and select for re-sistance to themselves and to other antibiotics. Even low doses of the drug help propagate resistant strains of bacteria, and these strains specify high levels of resistance. Besides the spread of the resistant bacteria among animals and from ani-mals to humans, the resistance determinants can be dissemi-nated via transposons or transferable plasmids to other bacte-ria that colonize people. In fact, the mobile DNA elements found in bacteria in animals are the very same ones found in human strains of the same bacteria.

Following the ban of antibiotics used for human health as growth promotants in animals in England, and later in a large part of Europe, other antibiotics were introduced for this pur-pose, including bacitracin, bambermycins, virginiamycin, and avoparcin. Some of these were already in use at the time. Ty-losan, a member of the macrolide antibiotic family (which in-cludes erythromycin and the newer broad-spectrum azithromycin and clarithromycin), was also a common feed additive in use since the early 1970s. Being active against gram-positive bacteria only, its promise, like that of virginia-mycin and avoparcin, was in impacting less on the general bacterial flora, especially the gram-negative bacteria. How-ever, a number of events removed the advantage, if any, of us-ing a narrower-spectrum growth promoter. For one, the gram-positive bacteria, including the enterococci, the staphy-lococci and the pneumococci, have reemerged as overriding causes of life-threatening human disease and antibiotic resis-tance is extremely prominent among these kinds of bacteria. Agents that treat the gram-positive bacteria have become more critical than ever to human therapy. In addition, only recently have we recognized the consequences of the struc-tural similarity of the growth promotant virginiamycin to the streptogramins (which make up the new human therapeutic

Synercid) and avoparcin to vancomycin. In fact, enterococci resistant to virginiamycin, which appeared in turkeys receiving virginiamycin, showed cross-resistance to *Synercid* via the same resistance mechanism.

Similarly, avoparcin, introduced as a growth promotant over 10 years ago, propagated strains of enterococci resistant to itself and to the structurally similar human-used antibiotic vancomycin. What was unforeseen when avoparcin was introduced was that a human analog, vancomycin, which represented less than .01% of all antibiotics prescribed in hospitals at the time, would become the essential last-resort drug for treating patients with hospital-borne MRSA in the 1990s. Thus, silently and unnoticed, the growth-promotant use of avoparcin has selected for avoparcin-resistant enterococci in animals, thus putting vancomycin's effectiveness for people at risk as well.

The world was first alerted to the connection between animals and vancomycin-resistant enterococci by Janice Bates and colleagues from Oxford, who discovered the vancomycin-resistant determinant among enterococci associated with small animals on one farm, with pigs on another farm, and even with retail-outlet chicken carcasses.[1] Vancomycin-resistant strains have been recovered from animals throughout Europe, where avoparcin has been used. Moreover, fecal carriage of vancomycin-resistant enterococci is relatively common in people living in countries where avoparcin is provided. In fact, recent studies show that humans associated with animals being fed avoparcin carry the same strains of enterococci as do their animals.

Ironically, while avoparcin has not been provided to animals in the U.S., the vancomycin-resistance problem is much larger in the U.S. today than in Europe. Individuals in the U.S. are not excreting vancomycin-resistant enterococci—except those who have returned from hospitals where they were prescribed the drug. The difference between Europe and the United States relates to how vancomycin is being used, compounded with the presence of the resistance determinant. In the U.S., the heavy use of vancomycin in hospitals for the treatment of MRSA or for diarrhea caused by *Clostridium difficile* selected and propagated the initially uncommon vancomycin-resistant enterococci now concentrated in hospitals. How the organism and resistance determinant came to the hospital is not known. They could have existed at low, undetectable levels in the hospitals and been subsequently selected by vancomycin use. Or, the strains could have arrived from areas of the world where avoparcin has been used for food production—crossing international borders with people or imported food.

While in a certain sense people in certain parts of Europe are living in a "sea" of vancomycin-resistant enterococci, the frequency of MRSA is low and vancomycin use in people is limited. Consequently, vancomycin resistance in hospital patients has been very low. The difference between the U.S. and Europe illustrates the local nature of resistance and the message from the so-called "antibiotic resistance equation" (Figure 6.1). Both the "antibiotic" and the "resistance determinant" are needed to produce a clinical resistance problem. Low human use of vancomycin in Europe has protected people from vancomycin resistance in the hospitals. However, from what we have learned in the U.S., as vancomycin usage increases in the European hospitals, the resistance determinant that resides there will become more prominent. The findings also predict the consequence and fate of so-called "animal-use only" drugs. A compound introduced as a growth promotant with no human benefit at one point in time can become a valued human therapeutic some 10–15 years later.

Animals and humans share in a large, interactive pool of susceptible and resistant bacteria containing movable resistance

Figure 6.1.   Antibiotic resistance equation—The emergence of a clinical antibiotic resistance problem requires the interaction of two major factors: the antibiotic that selects and the resistance gene being selected. If either is not present, a resistance problem will not exist.

determinants (Figure 6.2, next page). Humans can pick up these resistant bacteria and resistance genes from animals in different ways. Farm workers can do so during everyday activities in contact with the animals. Consumers do so by eating contaminated foods, especially those that are uncooked. A common scenario is the cook who uses the same kitchen counter surface to cut and season the meat and prepare the salads. While bacteria on the meat are killed during cooking, the salad retains the bacterial contamination and can even generate increased bacterial numbers if left to sit over a period of time.

   Pickup of resistance genes and bacteria from animals can occur indirectly through the use of animal manure as fertilizer. The resistant bacteria in the feces are tilled into the soil or sprayed onto the field. There they multiply and are retained during the harvest. Despite washing, these and other bacteria remain attached to the food crop and enter the consumer's

Figure 6.2. *This rendition of a quiet environmental scene belies the extensive activity going on at the microscopic level. In fact, bacteria and other microorganisms are multiplying, metabolizing, and exchanging genes. Transfer of bacterial hosts, their plasmids, and their genes is occurring among all participants of interactive environments throughout the world, including people, animals, fish, birds, insects, and plants (Bonnie Marshall, Tufts University School of Medicine).*

kitchen. One Dutch study followed bacteria from animals to the food chain, then into people, and finally to the sewers.

Farm workers who are in contact with animals have high levels of resistant bacteria in their normal intestinal flora. These resistant strains may have come from animals or may have been selected and propagated by the antibiotic being used. Bacteria can enter the human body through the mouth, nose, or throat and are swallowed, thus gaining access to the intestinal tract. While some of the bacteria harbored by animals will not colonize humans, it has been documented that a good number can and will. Since we are speaking of normal, harmless intestinal bacteria, the presence of resistance is of no immediate concern for farm workers. Moreover, there is no evidence that these workers have more disease than their counterparts working without antibiotics.

The issue is not disease incidence, but disease treatment. There are examples of farm workers or their families coming down with diseases that are hard to treat because of antibiotic resistance. For instance, one outbreak of resistant salmonellosis in a hospital newborn nursery in Connecticut in 1976 was traced to an infected calf on a nearby farm. The mother of the first infected infant came from that farm and was the presumed human source of the nursery infection.

More recently a cephalosporin-resistant *Salmonella*, the cause of severe illness in a young boy on a farm, was traced back to the animals on the farm, where use of a cephalosporin was the presumptive selective pressure for the emergence of this kind of resistance. While the antibiotic may have been used therapeutically, not subtherapeutically, the finding presents yet another example of the impact of animal use of antibiotics on resistant bacteria that can pass from animals to people.

Several experimental studies have brought to light some important facts relating to animal-human bacterial exchange. In the mid-1970s, my laboratory group examined the effect of subtherapeutic levels of a tetracycline antibiotic when introduced into a farm environment. We began with 300 chickens, just hatched from their eggs, that were delivered to a farm in Sherborn, Massachusetts. After initial rearing with heat lamps and a protective covering (Figure 6.3A, next page), the month-old chickens were divided and placed into six different cages for the experiment. Four cages were kept inside a barn; two were placed outside. About 50 chickens were placed in each cage, with males and females equally represented (Figure 6.3B).

One half of the chickens received feed containing subtherapeutic amounts (200 g/ton) of the antibiotic oxytetracycline. Over the course of nine months, we examined the feces of the

Figure 6.3. A) Newly hatched chickens were reared under heat lamps during the first weeks of life. B) Fifty adult chickens were placed in cages with equal numbers of males and females. The chickens in half the cages were fed with oxytetracycline-supplemented feed; the other half received normal feed.

oxytetracycline-fed and control groups of chickens, as well as the farm workers and family living in the farmhouse about 200 feet away. We also enlisted the help of neighboring families whose children attended the same schools. These people provided weekly stool samples for analysis. They acted as controls for any changes in bacterial flora not attributable to the chickens that might occur over the time period being examined.

Within 24–36 hours of feeding the oxytetracycline-laced feed to the chickens, their intestinal *Escherichia coli* were converted from susceptible to mostly resistant to tetracycline. Over the ensuing three months, other changes occurred. *E. coli* began to appear with resistance not only to tetracycline but also to ampicillin, streptomycin, and sulfonamides, even though the chickens had never been fed these drugs. In fact, no one had used these drugs on the farm at all.

Gradually, after five to six months, increased resistance appeared in the intestinal *E. coli* of the farm family members. One-third of the weekly fecal samples showed that almost all the *E. coli* were resistant to tetracycline. Moreover, by the sixth month, the *E. coli* carried resistance to four to five different antibiotics. The same phenomenon of multiple resistance that appeared in the chickens appeared to be emerging in the intestinal flora of farm inhabitants as time of tetracycline use on the farm lengthened, even though the people were *not* taking the tetracycline, nor were they eating the chickens. The intestinal flora of their neighbors, used as a control group, had none of these changes.

The study showed that these relatively small amounts of antibiotic could change the intestinal flora of animals and, more surprisingly, the flora of people living on the same farm. Clearly, antibiotics have an environmental effect. Moreover, chronic use of the drug (for two to three months) led to the emergence of bacteria with resistance to more than one antibiotic.

The appearance of multiple resistance from ingesting a single antibiotic is not unique to this study, or to chickens. It has been observed in other animals and in humans taking a single antibiotic for long periods of time. As noted earlier, women being treated with tetracycline for weeks for urinary tract infections were found to harbor bacteria in their intestines with resistance to many different antibiotics besides tetracycline. Patients taking long-term tetracycline or erythromycin to control acne were shown to harbor many different types of skin bacteria, all bearing resistance to three to six different antibiotics. In all cases, the emergence of multiple resistance followed chronic usage of only one antibiotic. The length of antibiotic usage influences the environmental microbial effect. Chronic use leads to multidrug resistance.

A group of studies during the mid- to late-1980s among pigs on farms in East Germany provided a different insight into the consequences of antibiotic use in animals and, in particular, to the spread of resistance. In this case, the transfer of a resistance determinant from animals to a whole neighboring human population was documented.

The investigators introduced a previously unused antibiotic, streptothricin, into the pigs' feed at levels intended for growth promotion. Before its introduction, no resistance to the drug could be found among bacteria associated with animals and humans, despite careful and quantitative measurements of fecal flora. Within six months of usage, however, a new resistance gene was discovered on transferable plasmids in the intestinal bacteria of the pigs. Of further importance, this resistance determinant was on a transposon, which explained why the resistance gene could be found on plasmids of various types in different intestinal bacteria.

Within two years, this resistance gene was recovered in 16–18% of all *E. coli* isolated from the feces of farm workers and their families as well as among people in the geographic area of the treated pigs. It also appeared in 1% of the bacteria causing urinary tract infections in this area. No streptothricin resistance was observed in people or animals in nearby areas where the antibiotic was not being used.

This rapid selection and spread revealed the extent of interaction between animal and human ecosystems. A resistance gene, selected in animals, entered human strains of *E. coli* and even strains causing human disease. Again, we are not saying that the bacteria are more infectious or will cause more disease. A resistance gene selected in animals can find its way into strains associated with humans. If it happened for the relatively unimportant streptothricin resistance gene, it could happen with others, such as those for resistance to penicillin, tetracyclines, and other human therapeutics. From an *E. coli* host, the resistance gene could eventually end up in bacteria causing disease.

Bonnie Marshall and other associates in my laboratory examined the natural spread of a resistant *E. coli* from one kind of animal to others and eventually to people. The experiment was designed to determine if *E. coli* harbored by one animal were somehow naturally confined to that animal. In other words, were there different kinds of *E. coli*, each specific to a particular kind of animal? We isolated an *E. coli* from a calf, marked it biochemically in the laboratory so that we could track it in the environment, and gave it back to the calf. The *E. coli* easily colonized the original calf, moved to mice in the same pen, and then moved to pigs, chickens and wild turkeys—all at significant distances away (Figure 6.4, next page). Of particular note, and probably linked to the spread, was the recovery of the marked organism from flies (caught on flypaper) at different locations in the barn. Human caretakers also began excreting these "calf" *E. coli*. The same phenomenon occurred with *E. coli* taken from pigs. The conclusion was clear. *E. coli* can colonize the intestines of many different kinds of animals. There-

166

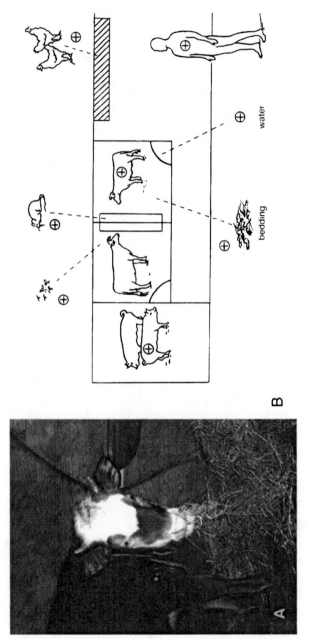

Figure 6.4. Spread of E. coli from an inoculated calf on a farm. An E. coli from the calf (A) was marked biochemically in the laboratory and re-fed to the animal. Over time, the "marked" E. coli could be recovered from other animate and inanimate objects in the barn (B) (Bonnie Marshall, Tufts University School of Medicine).

fore, there is no safeguard in the fact that the resistant bacteria selected by animal use of antibiotics emerge in the animals. These *E. coli* are environmental; their hosts may be many different animals—including people.

Transfer can occur in the opposite direction as well, that is, from humans to animals. In a study among baboons in Amboseli National Park in Kenya in 1982, investigators found significantly greater numbers of resistant bacteria in those animals eating human refuse from nearby campers than in their counterparts who lived on the natural diet in the wild (Figure 6.5, next page). On examination of the fecal flora, the animals feeding on human garbage had a flora strikingly similar to that of humans—diverse numbers of different *E. coli* with various sized plasmids. In contrast, baboons from the wild had flora showing a more harmonious group of *E. coli*, and only a small number of plasmids.

Animal-to-Human Spread of Disease-Causing Resistant Bacteria Through Food

In the last two decades, bacterial diseases from contaminated food have increased in the United States, leading to more sickness, hospitalizations, and even deaths. The infectious microorganism in most cases has been *Salmonella*, followed by *Campylobacter*. Both organisms can cause severe diarrhea. If the bacteria get into the bloodstream and multiply, they cause septicemia, characterized by high fevers and often death.

Salmonella and *Campylobacter* are commonly found in animals, where they can often be carried as a harmless commensal or one causing low-grade infection. In the 1980s, a number of outbreaks of *Salmonella* infections from food or milk occurred. Moreover, while *Salmonella* strains were uniformly susceptible to antibiotics prior to 1970, these incidents were caused by *Salmonella* resistant to at least two, if not four or

Figure 6.5. *Baboons feeding on human refuse placed in pits near campsites in Amboseli Park in Kenya. These baboons had a higher frequency of antibiotic resistance in their fecal flora than did their counterparts living in the wild.*

five, different antibiotics. In 1981, an outbreak of salmonellosis traced to one brand of precooked roast beef occurred in New Jersey and Pennsylvania and involved about one hundred people who contracted severe diarrhea. The microorganism was multiply resistant.

Investigations by members of the Centers for Disease Control and Prevention in Atlanta, Georgia, showed that such outbreaks caused by multiresistant *Salmonella* are increasing. Significantly, antibiotic ingestion by people is an important contributing factor to this increase. If infecting *Salmonella* are resistant, the chance of infection is higher in the people eating the contaminated product if they are also taking antibiotics (for some other reason) to which the *Salmonella* are insensitive. The resistant strain has an advantage when antibiotics are present since smaller numbers are sufficient to take hold in the body and cause disease. Other people, who are not taking an antibiotic but are eating the same contaminated product, might never get the disease because the numbers of infecting bacteria are too low. Had contaminating *Salmonella* microorganisms been susceptible to the antibiotic, this selection would not have taken place.

Another study in 1983 from the Centers for Disease Control traced a *Salmonella newport* outbreak in four Midwestern states to hamburger meat made from cattle from a single farm. Epidemiologic data showed that 12 of the 18 stricken individuals had been taking antibiotics to which the microorganism was resistant. The first thought of the CDC workers was that the antibiotic preparation was contaminated but, in fact, the antibiotic source of each individual had been different. What was common to each patient was that they had all eaten hamburger meat in the week before they got sick. This meat was traced to beef cattle from one farm in South Dakota adjoining a farm where a *Salmonella* of the same type had been isolated. The *Salmonella* were the same not only by type but also by the particular multiresistance plasmid that they contained. Putting the pieces of the puzzle together, the CDC epidemiologists concluded that the likely route of infection was from beef cattle, to the meat in processing plants, to the packages in the grocery stores. Again, the concentration of *Salmonella* in the meat was assessed to have been small; hence, many people who ate the hamburger meat were unaffected. Those who were taking antibiotics to which the *Salmonella* were resistant, however, provided a perfect environment for the resistant strain to multiply, leading to overt clinical disease.

In 1985 in California, several hundred individuals who developed diarrhea had *Salmonella newport* isolated from their diarrheal specimens. The source for disease in all these individuals was again hamburger meat. Two people died. The investigators traced the microorganism, identified by its plasmid, to dairy cattle, where it could still be isolated. The microorganism was also found in the processing plants and in the remaining unsold meat. Besides using therapeutic antibiotics, the farmer was also feeding subtherapeutic amounts of penicillin and tetracycline to the animals. The *Salmonella* were resistant to the subtherapeutic and therapeutic drugs used on that farm. This was the first definitive study, using biochemical and microbiological techniques, that traced the causative microorganism from an animal source to humans via all parts of the food chain.

Milk has also been a source of *Salmonella* infections. One outbreak in 1987 in Arizona occurred from raw milk and was traced back to infected animals. One of the largest outbreaks of *Salmonella* infection linked to milk occurred in northern Illinois in the spring of 1985 and affected people in three other states. A total of 200,000 people contracted the disease from packaged milk. Again, studies showed that the antibacterial resistance of the strain increased its attack rate, since, among the infected people, a larger than normal percentage was taking an antibiotic for some reason. This antibiotic ingestion put them at greater risk. Again, the culprit microorganism was multiresistant. The milk, two different brands of pasteurized 2% milk from a single dairy, became contaminated apparently through a leakage in the system that mixed raw milk with pasteurized milk.

These studies should leave no question that domestic food animals can be a source of resistant bacterial infections in humans. Since food animals are routinely and chronically being fed antibiotics, the microorganisms that they harbor are often multiply resistant, a situation that produces an additional health hazard to the human population. Paradoxically, being multiresistant, the bacteria pose a greater potential problem to those *already* taking an antibiotic for another illness. While there is less use of antibiotics for growth promotion in the cattle industry than in the swine industry, the beef industry has been the most common source of resistant infections. This finding is largely linked to many people's tastes for rare beef, and cooking does not kill all the bacteria associated with the raw meat. Only infrequently does meat other than beef get ground up for hamburger, mixing the exposed outer surfaces with the inner tissues. Swine and poultry are generally well cooked, thus killing off any contaminating bacteria.

We may wonder how the subtherapeutic use of drugs can still work effectively. Given the years of usage, one would expect that the antibiotic has selected countless resistant strains. We may also wonder which drugs can be used effectively when these animals get sick.

There are indications that resistance *has* become a problem when trying to treat animals that have been taking subtherapeutic amounts of antibiotics. New drugs are being used to treat illnesses in these animals that were previously controlled by the older line of antibiotics. Resistance was presumably the reason that the farmer caring for the dairy cows on the farm in California where subtherapeutic doses of penicillin and tetracycline were given had to use the restricted and illegal antibiotic chloramphenicol to treat his sick cows. The other appropriate antibiotics were useless in the face of resistance. Even in this case, chloramphenicol was ineffective, since these *Salmonella* also bore resistance to the drug—a resistance seen infrequently in clinical strains of bacteria in the United States.

Fluoroquinolones became needed for animal treatment when infectious organisms appeared with resistance to other drugs. In the 1990s, strains of *Salmonella typhimurium* emerged with resistance to fluoroquinolones, one of the few drugs left to treat this multidrug-resistant organism. The appearance occurred shortly after the introduction of fluoroquinolones as therapy for animals. The multidrug-resistant *Salmonella typhimurium* strain DT104, resistant to five or more antibiotics, appeared in animals in the United Kingdom, the U.S., and elsewhere. It was later linked to disease in people.

In the past decade, investigators in Holland reported a temporal association between the use of fluoroquinolones in chickens and a rise in fluoroquinolone-resistant *Campylobacter* causing diarrhea in people. More recently, in the state of Minnesota, epidemiologists discovered that the introduction of fluoroquinolones for the treatment of poultry led to an increase in fluoroquinolone-resistant *Campylobacter jejuni* in people traced to the chickens. This finding led the Center for Veterinary Medicine (U.S. Food and Drug Administration) in 2000 to propose a ban on the use of fluoroquinolones as treatment, the first time the agency has taken such a decisive action. Although not accepted by the industry, the proposal is under close evaluation by the FDA, other U.S. agencies, industry, and public interest groups.

What can be done and what should be done? Many farmers believe that they need these antibiotics in order to raise healthy and hardy animals. This may or may not be true, depending on how the animals are raised and the conditions of the farm, as well as the number of animals being housed together. Certainly, the close confinement practices of some large farm complexes set the stage for cross-contamination with infectious diseases. This is presumably the reason why, in the raising of veal cattle, the milk fed to them is almost uniformly supplemented with tetracycline.

Even though any proposed legislative action to eliminate subtherapeutic use of antibiotics in animal feeds has been delayed in congress for over 25 years, the situation is not completely dormant. There is increasing pressure from individuals and public interest groups to limit this type of usage. Mounting evidence has revealed the resistance problem. There is a growing understanding that these valuable human antibiotics are not needed or even useful for promoting growth of animals. The poultry industry, which once used penicillins and tetracyclines universally for growth promotion, claims that only about 20% or less of producers do so now.

The Center for Veterinary Medicine of the U.S. Food and Drug Administration has introduced a Framework Document to deal formally with this issue. In short, the document categorizes antibiotics based on their importance to human health. For instance, those drugs that are extremely useful to human care would not be permitted for use as growth promotants and would be restrained from any animal use unless no other therapeutic options were available. Two other categories contain drugs with little or no importance to human health. The document represents an important focus for discussion of this critical issue by regulators, consumer action groups, microbiologists, and industry.

Following public concern about the problem of resistant salmonellosis traced to beef, the Cattlemen's Association advised its constituents to stop using antibiotics for growth promotion of beef cattle. It asked that drugs not used in humans, ones other than antibiotics, be the only ones added to the animal feed. Today, this practice is largely followed. Monensin, an animal-use-only chemical, is a successful alternative. Recently, limits in antibiotic use for growth have been advocated by the swine industry as well.

New and old alternatives for penicillins and tetracyclines are available for growth promotion. Bacitracins, which are nonabsorbable antibiotics not used for internal human infections but only for local skin lesions, were shown, even in the early 1950s, to produce a growth-promotion effect. Some of the early data showed that bacitracin had an effect equal to that of tetracycline. Today bacitracins continue to be used successfully in animal husbandry. In the chicken industry, bacitracins or the bambermycins, another group of nonabsorbable antimicrobials, are the growth-promoting agents principally used. This change is a major step forward.

Growth-promotant practice has been eliminated in Sweden and Denmark. In the European Union, a number of growth-promotant antibiotics, including avoparcin, virginiamycin, spiramycin, and tylosin, were officially banned at the end of the last decade, with a consequent drop in sales as expected. This action was made on the "precautionary principle," in view of the fact that the drugs can select for bacteria bearing resistance to antibiotics of human need. While virginiamycin and tylosin are still used in the United States, avoparcin has never been used there. Still, the practice of providing penicillins and tetracyclines for growth continues in the United States. The FDA Framework Document should have a positive impact if it will affect use of the older antibiotics as well as the new ones.

An historic event occurred at a meeting convened by the World Health Organization in October 1997 in Berlin, Germany. A large number of representatives from industry, government, and academia met to discuss the human health impact of antibiotic use in animals. The meeting was preceded by an electronic discussion, one of the first of its kind, that focused on the issue. Invited experts posted their papers on the website and then attendees and others throughout the world discussed and debated the viewpoints. At the meeting in October, several important points were made by various parties. From the U.S. Centers for Disease Control and Prevention came the argument that all *Salmonella* resistance had emerged among animals, since over 90% of the cases of *Salmonella* are spread through animal sources. Whether this resistance emerged through therapeutic or subtherapeutic use was not viewed as an important point; animals were accepted as the source of the resistant *Salmonella*. An important example was the emergence and spread of the multidrug-resistant *Salmo-*

nella typhimurium DT104 from animals to people, which we discussed earlier. The group endorsed more appropriate therapeutic use. For the first time, data were presented on the problem posed by antibiotics used only for animals, which were not obvious human therapeutics at the time they were first implemented. For example, avoparcin and virginiamycin, considered "animal-only" antibiotics, could select strains resistant to drugs recently approved for humans. This understanding led the attendees to agree that any use of an antibiotic in animals could eventually impact human health needs, even decades later when some chemical modification converted an animal-use drug into one useful for human therapy. The attendees reinforced the resolution that any antimicrobial that is used in human therapy or that can select for resistance to a human therapeutic should not be used in growth promotion. But the biggest achievement of the meeting, and that which makes it historic, was the passing of the recommendation to replace growth-promotant use of antibiotics entirely.

> Increased concerns regarding risks to public health resulting from the use of antimicrobial growth promoters indicate that it is essential to have a systematic approach towards replacing growth-promoting antimicrobials with safer non-antimicrobial alternatives.[2]

Clearly the world was preparing itself for the eventual removal of antibiotics as subtherapeutic agents for growth promotion. The examples of virginiamycin and avoparcin poignantly illustrated the problem at hand. While these drugs were not for human use when they were introduced in the 1970s for growth promotion, these compounds are the chemical basis for human therapeutics needed to fight newly emergent infections. Any antibiotic provided to animals will produce an environment of resistant organisms, which can cause imminent resistance problems when a structurally-related drug is introduced for human use.

As we enter a new decade, there is increased optimism that advances will be made to control the use of subtherapeutic amounts of antibiotics for growth promotion.

The veterinary profession itself has seen the problems and discrepancies between the availability of antibiotics to live-stock owners and the availability to humans. Summarizing their view of veterinary medicine in the 21st century, William Pritchard and Frank Loew described the freer access of ani-mal owners than of laypeople to a multitude of potent antimi-crobials. This is also true of livestock owners as compared to pet owners. They estimate that "approximately 93% of the drugs approved for animals can be used by livestock owners without veterinary supervision."[3] They see the public's con-cern about the "environmental issues raised by these practices and by the potential for contamination of foods with residues and pathogens." They suggest that veterinarians should play active roles in finding ways to reduce the "risks entailed with such widespread use of potent antimicrobials." Veterinarians are certainly an important group to rally for action.

A consortium of environmental advocacy groups, includ-ing the Union of Concerned Scientists, the Environmental Defense Fund, and the Center for Science in the Public In-terest, joined together in 2000 to demand the end of growth-promotant use of antibiotics on the basis of adverse environmental effects and a threat to human health. The in-ternational *Alliance for the Prudent Use of Antibiotics* orga-nized a project called FAAIR (Facts about Antibiotic use in Animals and its Impact on Resistance), which examined the broad ecological consequences of antibiotic use in animals. Its document, released in 2001, tracks antibiotic use in ani-mals to various ecological areas and environments (Figure

6.6, next page). This project involved a multidisciplinary group of experts who examined the science behind the environmental impact of animal use of antibiotics and revealed the broad extent of antibiotic transport and consequences to ecology. The group concluded that antibiotics provided to animals and agriculture contribute to the global environment pool of antimicrobial resistance genes and resistant bacteria. Given that a considerable amount of antimicrobials is used in animals and the fact that bacteria and resistance genes exchange among animals and people, the group strongly recommended reduction in the non-therapeutic use of antimicrobials in farm animals and agriculture. They also urged caution in the use of new generation antibiotics, namely, cephalosporins and fluoroquinolones, in animals. They predicted that such efforts would lower the amount of antimicrobial resistance in the environment, leading to beneficial effects on human and animal health. However, attention to resistance stemming from animal use is not meant to deny the major influence of antibiotic misuse in people on the resistance problem in humans. The focus on animals runs parallel to that in people, with additional emphasis on the wide ecologic effect of animal use.

The outcry from animal rights groups about the crowded conditions for raising animals and the concern shown by microbiologists and clinicians about emergent resistant strains have led to renewed interest in raising animals in the traditional way. "Natural food farms" have begun to proliferate in New York State and in many parts of the Midwest. These farms claim to produce an excellent product without reliance on chemical or antibiotic food additives. The Chicago-based Food Animal Concerns Trust (FACT), a nonprofit, publicly financed organization, promotes farms that raise animals under conditions where antibiotic supplementation is not given. The group supported the Rambling Rose brand of veal for

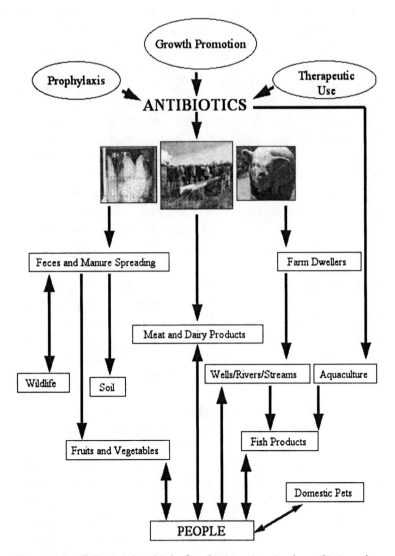

Figure 6.6. *Following three kinds of antibiotic use in animals, antibiotics and antibiotic-resistant bacteria enter wide environmental niches, and can eventually come in contact with and impact people. (Designed by APUA, Boston, MA, www.apua.org)*

some time. This veal was produced from nonanemic calves raised outdoors and fed non-antibiotic-supplemented milk containing iron and nutrients. Farms were located in New York, Pennsylvania, and Texas. While the meat was pink and not white like that of the anemic calf, a small but sustained market for the product appeared because of the meat's good taste and quality. Some of the finer restaurants in New York, Chicago, and San Francisco boasted the Rambling Rose mark on their menus, including Chanterelle in New York. Because of problems in distribution, this project was discontinued in 1991, but the experiment was successful in showing that it could be done and that the product had a market.

In 1984, FACT launched its first chicken egg product, called Nest Eggs, which was sold throughout the New York, northern New Jersey, and Chicago areas. The hens are raised on farms in Illinois, Pennsylvania, and New Jersey, where they are free to roam in straw litter, not crowded in cages. FACT has shown that this alternative measure for raising animals is profitable and successful.

Moreover, the "free-range" chickens are monitored to maintain low levels, if any, of *Salmonella* in the eggs. Through ongoing research, the group aims to prove that more "humane" farming methods produce safer, commercially profitable eggs.

Groups such as the National Resources Defense Council have attempted legal action to get the United States Food and Drug Administration Center for Veterinary Medicine to ban the use of human antibiotics in animal feeds. The efforts have not been legislatively successful but have brought the issues to the public where consumers are heeding the call.

A number of new approaches are being tried to control infectious diseases and/or increase growth and so avoid the use of antibiotics. One deals with "competitive exclusion"—bacteria of one sort are given to the animal as a means to exclude others. This is the rationale behind the product *Preempt*, containing 29 non-pathogenic bacterial strains from the fecal contents of an adult hen, which is sprayed onto newly hatched chicks to prevent colonization by *Salmonella*. This exclusion approach was championed in the 1970s by Dr. Esko Nurmi from Finland, who fed baby chicks a mixture of bacteria from the intestinal tract of adult hens and showed that they were protected from *Salmonella* infection. Another recent product marketed for poultry, called *Ovation*, is a powder that contains antibodies to cholecystokinin, an intestinal peptide that causes food to move rapidly in the intestinal tract. The antibody inhibits the peptide, thus causing normal, slower movement and increased availability of nutrients, which leads to growth promotion without the need for antibiotics.

Optimistically, the combined efforts of livestock owners, veterinarians, and consumers can lead to a change in the use of human therapeutics as growth enhancers in large livestock production. If consumers hold out for more naturally raised products, the producers will inevitably deliver it. Given legislative politics, better-educated consumers will demand products from animals not raised on antibiotics needed for human treatment. Only then will we see definitive changes in this area of antibiotic usage.

chapter seven

Further Ecologic Considerations

*Antibiotic Use in Agriculture,
Aquaculture, Pets, and Minor Animal Species*

The bulk of antibiotics produced in the United States treats human infections and promotes growth and controls infections in food animals. Many of the same drugs, however, have found their places in the treatment of diseases affecting pets, such as dogs and cats, as well as trees, plants, fish, and even honeybees.

Poultry, cattle, and pigs represent the largest group of animals being raised for food consumption, members of what the United States Food and Drug Administration calls the "major species" of animals, which also includes horses, dogs, and cats. Other food animals raised in lesser numbers, such as lambs, sheep, and goats, which are members of the "minor species," likewise receive antibiotics. So do fish and animals raised for their pelts, such as mink. Compared with the estimated 40–50 million pounds of antibiotics given annually in the United

States to the major food animals and to humans, the total amount of antibiotics given yearly to these other animals and used for agriculture is relatively small. It probably accounts for only about half a million pounds. The impact of this use on the environment, namely, in the selection of resistant bacteria, however, may still be considerable.

Antibiotic Use in Agriculture

Bacteria and other microbial agents cause diseases in plants and trees. It is, therefore, not surprising to find that antibiotics can control and treat some of these diseases. To get the antibiotic to each plant or tree, however, broad-scale methods are often needed. Although some antibiotics can be injected into tree trunks, today tree farm owners generally treat by spraying antibiotics onto the affected plants and trees. This approach is used chiefly to control infections known to be present or to prevent ones from entering at a particularly vulnerable growth period. As a result, this mode of drug delivery enlarges the potential ecological consequences of antibiotics since application is to an area, not to a single infected host plant. As with other antibiotic treatments, this use on field crops leads to the killing of susceptible bacteria inhabiting that environment, as well as the pathogens under treatment. In a perverse way, therefore, even though these are comparatively small amounts of antibiotics, they have a potentially significant effect *vis-a-vis* the selection of resistant bacteria. Depending on the scale of dispersal, this usage can be an important contributor to the emergence of resistance in bacteria sharing the environment with human beings.

Two antibiotics, oxytetracycline and streptomycin, are currently registered in the United States for use in the treatment of diseases of trees and plants. This registration dates back about 50 years—to the decade of the discovery of these drugs and their successful use in humans. Today, in the United

States, about 100,000 pounds of antibiotics are used each year just for the control of bacterial infections of fruit trees. One pound (about 450 grams) is enough antibiotic for one day's treatment of 450 people.

Originally discovered in 1943, streptomycin became popular in treating agricultural plant diseases in 1952. Although used more extensively in the 1950s and 1960s, it still holds its own as a common treatment today. For instance, streptomycin is generally applied to mitigate "soft rot" or "black leg" in potatoes (Figure 7.1, next page). These bacterial diseases cause decay of the growing potato tuber. It is also used for the treatment of "wild fire" or "blue mold" of tobacco plant seed beds. These are also bacterial diseases that begin in breaks in the leaf and end up killing the plants. Likewise, to prevent "bacterial blight" on celery during the transplanting of seedlings, and to protect peppers and tomatoes from "bacterial spot," streptomycin has become a standard treatment.

Oxytetracycline is a form of the more commonly used tetracycline. It is less easily absorbed into the human body and for this reason has found its place in treating surfaces of animals and plants where absorption into the body is not needed for its activity. For instance, this form of tetracycline is used to treat bacteria in the intestinal tracts of food animals. It is also effective when injected into certain tree roots or trunks to treat bacterial infection.

The species of bacteria that cause diseases in animals and plants are different from those causing infections in humans. These bacteria have features similar to bacteria that cause diseases in humans, however, and may be distantly related. They belong to common *families* consisting of multiple types or species that share certain characteristics, although each of the members may show a propensity to infect different human, animal, or plant hosts. For instance, many bacterial agents of plant diseases are classified as mycoplasma or mycoplasmalike. The plant mycoplasma is different from the *Mycoplasma*

Figure 7.1.   *Antibiotics, chiefly streptomycin and oxytetracycline, are used to control bacterial infections of fruits and vegetables (Bonnie Marshall, Tufts University School of Medicine).*

pneumoniae that causes respiratory tract infections in humans, but they share certain likenesses. They are bacteria that do not have complete cell walls nor the capacity to synthesize them. Because of this feature, they are naturally resistant to antibiotics that affect cell wall synthesis, such as penicillins, but are sensitive to those that affect protein synthesis, such as tetracycline, chloramphenicol, and erythromycin. While not known, it is possible that genetic material, such as resistance genes, could be exchanged between the plant and animal mycoplasma. While only distantly related, the similarities between these kinds of bacteria affecting animals and plants may still be more than that shared by gram-positive and gram-negative bacteria known to exchange resistance genes.

Erwinia is a primary target group for antibiotics in the treatment of fruit tree diseases. Members of this genus belong to the

Enterobacteriaceae, the same family that includes *Escherichia coli*, *Salmonella*, and *Shigella*. Bacteria in this family can exchange genes among themselves, including plant pathogens. Apple and pear trees are the most important victims of *Erwinia amylovora*, which causes a disease known as "fire blight"—a withering of the leaves and decaying of fruit. The microorganism enters the trees through wounds in the flower or leaf and then moves to other parts of the tree. Streptomycin appears to be the drug of choice in combating *Erwinia*. In certain areas, however, resistance to streptomycin has appeared in *Erwinia*, making streptomycin ineffective. This event has necessitated a change to oxytetracycline, which is, fortunately, effective. Oxytetracycline is likewise efficient in controlling blemishes, or "bacterial spots," on peaches caused by another gram-negative bacteria, *Xanthomonas*. Applications are generally done by airblast spraying from movable apparatuses pulled by trucks through the rows of trees.

The application of antibiotics to fruit trees occurs throughout the United States, but chiefly on the two coasts. In the western coastal states of Washington, Oregon, and California, primarily pear and apple trees are treated, while antibiotic treatment in the East involves mostly peach and apple trees. Antibiotic application usually begins at the first suspicion or sign of a disease problem.

At the end of the last decade, principally nine states were using oxytetracycline on their fruit trees: New Jersey, Maryland, North Carolina, South Carolina, Georgia, Missouri, Michigan, Illinois, and Indiana. Of the total acreage devoted to growing pear and peach trees in the United States at that time, about 25–30% of the pear crop areas (occupying some 20,000 acres) and 15% (about 15,000 acres) of the peach areas received treatments. Today, the situation is similar. This is not much, considering the vast size of the United States, but could produce significant changes in the bacterial flora of these treatment sites and the people living there.

Aerial spraying by airblasts from the ground and occasionally by airplanes (this latter method having declined in recent years) results in antibiotic application to areas outside those specified for treatment. Dusting, such as on potatoes, and hand-held sprayers allow homeowners and gardeners to treat their own plants and fruit trees with a greater degree of confinement. Both applications, however, potentially affect more than the immediate environment. With dusting, the user's own intestinal and skin flora may be "treated," since small amounts of antibiotics can be ingested or deposited on the skin.

For this reason, antibiotic use in agriculture is under strict regulation by the U.S. Environmental Protection Agency. Providers must wear clothing, boots, gloves, and masks in mixing and applying the antibiotics to the designated areas. Besides the national laws, individual states may have regulations that further help protect the antibiotic deliverers and the environment from substantial antibiotic contact. Still, it is evident that an antibiotic being applied in this way is hard to control, even under the best conditions.

Antibiotics are applied on other types of vegetation besides fruit trees. Antibiotics exert a beneficial effect by delaying or controlling "lethal yellowing," a mycoplasmalike infection of ornamental palms, coconut palms, date palms, and others. In the 1970s in Miami, 40,000 coconut palms were affected, and 75% of those in Dade County were killed. Oxytetracycline by injection is the drug of choice for the problem and is used mainly in Florida and Texas.

Among ornamental plants, chrysanthemums are treated by placing cuttings directly into an antibiotic solution in order to protect them against bacterial diseases. Dieffenbachia, philodendron, and pyracantha are often treated with antibiotics for bacterial diseases that lead to withering of the leaves, or so-called "fire blight." As in all plant applications, the aim of treatment is prevention, since no cure is attainable in plants once they become diseased. Therefore, it is important for the grower to know exactly during which growth stages plants are most likely to contract disease.

During the 1950s, when streptomycin was being used on fruit trees, the United States Food and Drug Administration examined the fruit for residues. Within the limits of detection (0.5 parts per million), no residues were found. This examination is still done periodically wherever treatments are applied, to assure that no residual antibiotic can be inadvertently ingested by the consumer. This safeguard is important; however, the long-term effect on the microbial ecology of an agricultural area, that is, the selection of resistant strains of bacteria, cannot be monitored so easily.

Although streptomycin is one of the two antibiotics applied to plants, it is rarely used today in human medicine because of the discovery of newer and less toxic agents. Streptomycin resistance, for some unknown reason, is among the most common resistances found in bacterial strains associated with people. However, some believe that this is the result of prior streptomycin selection followed by continued propagation, despite the absence of the antibiotic. Curiously, streptomycin resistance rarely occurs alone; it is generally found in conjunction with other resistance determinants. Therefore, while streptomycin resistance per se may have little consequence on human therapy today, when streptomycin is used, it selects not only bacteria with streptomycin resistance but also those bearing resistance to other useful antibiotics. In this way, the environmental pool of multidrug resistance is widened. Certain *Erwinia amylovora* have been isolated with multidrug resistance on transferable plasmids. From the standpoint of agriculture, streptomycin or tetracycline resistance, when it occurs, seriously thwarts plant therapy, since few approved alternative antibiotics are available.

The heyday of antibiotic treatment of plants and trees was in the 1950s during the height of antibiotic discovery. But as time passed, the disease-causing microorganisms began to appear resistant to the very drugs being used to kill them—just as we have seen in the treatment of humans. Clinicians, microbiologists, and veterinarians also began to raise health concerns about the residues left on food produce. In response to these concerns, other means of disease control, such as nonantibiotic chemical treatments, began to replace the use of antibiotics. Not all substitute measures, however, could supplant antibiotics. Some disease agents could not be managed any other way. Therefore, streptomycin and oxytetracycline are still important agents in treating certain susceptible bacterial diseases of fruit and agricultural crops. Guarding the susceptibility of this population must be a goal, given the already high frequency of resistance to these antibiotics in other bacteria in the environment. As in other areas, therefore, misuse and particularly prolonged use should be avoided.

The major problem we are addressing here is not antibiotic residues on or in food produce, but rather the enormous selection that even small amounts of these agents can have for resistant bacteria. In the wake of killing susceptible bacteria, resistant forms, even rare ones, emerge, propagate, and can predominate in the treated area. There are no present-day tests for measuring the frequency of these resistant bacteria. They could someday be a problem to agriculture. They could also have wider consequences. If they find their way into the vicinity of bacteria that colonize the gut or the skin of people or animals, they could pass their resistance traits to these bacterial strains. In this way, resistance traits selected in agriculture could be spread to humans.

In 1996, Quimica Agronomica in Mexico, wishing to export apples to the U.S., requested EPA permission to allow residues of gentamicin on apples at 0.1 parts per million. The Public and Scientific Affairs Board of the 42,000-member American Society for Microbiology wrote a firm letter against the allowance of gentamicin sulfate in or on apples at any concentration. Drs. Gail Cassell, chair of the Board, and Anne Vidaver, chair of the

Committee on Agricultural Food and Industry, stressed that gentamicin was critical in treating a variety of bacteria causing human disease such as septicemia, burn wounds, peritonitis, appendicitis, and other abdominal infections. The letter stated that the use of gentamicin would directly and indirectly expose resident microorganisms to the antibiotic, with a high possibility of selecting drug-resistant organisms—especially troublesome would be those with transferable resistance. Moreover, if this practice were done in the United States, the workers would have been protected by strict guidelines, as we discussed. There was no evidence of any such practice in Mexico nor any attempt to examine the Mexican orchard workers. The issue was also politically hot. The State Department was notified because refusal of importation threatened the NAFTA treaty between the United States and Mexico. The letter and those from other groups had impact on the EPA decision and the request appears to be still on hold. As an event, it demonstrates the consequence of a seemingly simple request when an agency and experts see the broader impact of antibiotic use via an effect on resistance development and a change in the microbial environment.

Contamination of crops with antibiotic-resistant microorganisms of more potential clinical relevance may occur by another route. Resistant fecal strains of bacteria can contaminate agricultural plots and their crops through the use of manure from antibiotic-fed animals. In certain areas of England, Europe, and the United States, conveyer belts move fecal slush from pigs or other animals out to agricultural lands where it is aerated and dispersed as a spray onto the growing agricultural plants. It is through this application that resistant bacteria could be transferred from animals to other ecosystems, in this case agricultural products. Studies have shown that birds feeding amongst the dispersed manure pick up and ingest these resistant microorganisms. Flies can carry fecal *Escherichia coli* for quite long distances. The full extent of this procedure's contribution to the general problem of antibiotic resistance in humans is not yet understood. Given our current situation with the enlarging pool of multiple antibiotic resistances, we should devote time to studying this area of potential antibiotic resistance spread.

How resistant bacteria actually travel through the food chain can be explained through various scenarios. Washing fruits or vegetables may clean off the dirt, but washing can cause a more thorough spread of existing bacteria. If a vegetable has leaves or crevices, bacteria can find their way into these or even into its interior. The outer leaves of lettuce are full of bacteria from the soil and from manure and other contacts with animals and humans. In contrast, the inner leaves are virtually clean. Unless lettuce is washed leaf by leaf, as the French people usually do, the bacteria from the outside leaves enter the inside ones. The removal of the pedicel from a tomato (plucked from the plant) leaves an opening to the inside of the fruit. Thus, bacteria may enter into the tomato where they find plenty of nutrients for growth and multiplication.

In studies of bacteria associated with fruits and vegetables from local food markets in Boston, we have found large numbers, 10,000 to 100,000, of antibiotic-resistant bacteria per gram of vegetable. These bacteria were not particularly harmful, but 10–20% of them were potentially able to colonize human intestines. While they were not disease-causing, these strains did carry resistance genes that could be transferred to other bacteria in laboratory experiments. In immunocompromised patients, such as those undergoing cancer chemotherapy, even these relatively harmless bacteria can result in disease. If resistant, they would be more difficult to treat. For instance, on market produce we found *Klebsiella* bacteria with multiple resistance on plasmids that were transferable to *Escherichia coli*, a natural member of our intestinal flora. While not usually harmful, *E. coli* becomes a reservoir for resistance traits that could give a person trouble later, especially in an immunocompromised state during cancer therapy. Recall, for example, the previously discussed patient who died from a multidrug-resistant *E. coli* while being treated for leukemia.

I once instructed hospital medical staff, during a learning exercise, to take a tomato, slice it with a sterile knife, and then place the slice for several seconds on top of agar that contained nutrients for growth. After the slice was removed, the plate was incubated overnight at body temperature (37°C or 98°F). The next day the complete image of the tomato slice was replicated on the plate, designed by colonies from the bacteria within the tomato. None of the bacteria were harmful—mostly soil types or those carried by humans and animals in our intestinal tracts. Further study, however, showed that about 10% of these bacteria were antibiotic resistant and, again, were the kinds that could colonize our intestinal tract.

On the basis of these studies and those performed by others elsewhere, uncooked fruits and vegetables are conventionally removed from the diets of patients undergoing therapy for cancer at a time when their host defense systems are suppressed and when common bacteria can take over and cause severe disease.

Antibiotic use in agriculture is varied. The applications are very different from those for antibiotics used in animals and humans. The environmental ramifications from even small doses can still be significant in the selection of resistant variants. Some of these may bear transferable resistance plasmids and transposons, bringing direct problems to the agricultural growers and potential changes to other microbial participants in our shared environment.

Antibiotic Use in Honeybees

American and European foulbrood diseases cause the death of countless honeybees and the consequent loss of hives. In the United States, oxytetracycline is the only antibiotic permitted for use in beehives. American foulbrood is caused by *Bacillus larvae*, a rod-shaped gram-positive bacterium; the European disease is caused by *Streptococcus pluton*, a gram-positive coccus. In general, the antibiotic is recommended only for preventing and controlling the disease from spreading from one infected hive to others in the vicinity of the infected hive. Some bee-keepers use this antibiotic for treatment of the infected hive itself, but this application has been vigorously debated. Some states have laws against it. Many believe that treatment of infected hives does not help the overall beehive situation. For one thing, it could lead to resistant bacteria and thus cause ineffective treatment if later infections arise. For another, once the bacteria, namely *B. larvae*, are established, it is hard, if not impossible, to get rid of them. Consequently, it is better to destroy the hive with the bacteria. There is also the possibility that infected hives could contain bees that are somehow more susceptible to infectious agents. Therefore, if these bees and their hives are salvaged, the effect would be to propagate hives that are more susceptible, not only to this foulbrood disease but also to other potential disease-causing agents.

Treatment is usually given in the early spring and fall, when there are few flowers in bloom. At this time, in the absence of nectar sources, the bees pick up the infection by scavenging honey from other infected hives. During those periods of potential infection, oxytetracycline is applied in powdered sugar directly to the hive. It is the larvae that must be protected. The adult bees, in the process of housekeeping, remove the antibiotic sugar mix and thus make contact with the tetracycline. It is then inadvertently delivered by them to their brood of larvae, which, in this way, receives protection from the infectious agents.

Some history of antibiotic use in bees is in order. In the early 1950s, other antibiotics such as sulfathiazole and streptomycin were used to treat foulbrood disease. Because these drugs did not work effectively, however, erythromycin, a different kind of antibiotic, was added. Then in 1955, in San Luis Valley, Colorado, beekeepers noted that the disease was suddenly not responding to erythromycin. This event, and other similar cases elsewhere, were among the first to alert beekeepers to the problem of bacterial resistance. The emergence of antibiotic-resistant bacteria contributed to the decision to destroy infected hives rather than to propagate weak hives and their resistant bacteria.

From the time that oxytetracycline was first introduced, honey was routinely examined for drug residues. None were found. According to an official in the Division of Beneficial Insects Laboratory of the United States Department of Agriculture, the reason is that the antibiotic is not stable and breaks down in the hive and in honey. This laboratory of the USDA also periodically checks for resistant *Bacillus* from among bacterial isolates sent to them from infected hives. Until now, no oxytetracycline resistance in the bacillus causing this disease has been found. This is indeed fortunate, since other members of the genus *Bacillus* are known to carry resistance to this antibiotic. By the present treatment method, oxytetracycline loses its effectiveness in the hive in less than ten days. Thus, it does not remain as a continued selective agent. This may be a reason for the yet-unseen problem of resistance to it. The application of oxytetracycline to control infection of honeybee larvae is not perceived as a particular contributor to environmental selection of antibiotic-resistant bacteria. My interest in describing this practice is to point out how diverse antibiotic usage is as an almost everyday happening. Moreover, it may be that in this limited area, careful use may be controlling a potential resistance problem. Certainly, if resistance should emerge, then preventive use of tetracyclines will have to be changed. Which alternative drugs will be as safe and as effective is unknown. It would be in the best interests of the beekeeper to continue to have tetracycline available as the drug of choice. In order to assure this present situation, the current use of tetracycline must remain appropriate, that is, given only when needed.

Antibiotic Use in Commercial Fish

Three antibiotics related to ones effective in human medicine are also used for the treatment of bacterial infections in salmon, catfish, trout, and other commercially raised fish. These antibiotics are oxytetracycline and Romet–30, a combination of sulfadimethoxine (a sulfonamide derivative) and ormetoprim (a derivative of trimethoprim). In particular, they are used to treat ulcers or furunculoses of the skin of the fish, as well as diarrhea and blood-borne sepsis. These infections are caused by rodlike gram-negative microorganisms belonging to bacterial families that also produce disease in humans. To ensure protection of the consumer against antibiotic residues, the United States Food and Drug Administration requires a withdrawal time before fish can be harvested and sold. Withdrawal times depend both on the antibiotic and on the fish. For instance, in catfish the withdrawal time for ormetoprim is 3 days, but for salmon it is 42 days. The withdrawal time for oxytetracycline is 21 to 30 days for all fish.

The antibiotic oxytetracycline is also used to protect American lobsters, held in "tidal pounds" in the United States and Canada, from gaffkemia (caused by *Aerococcus viridans*), a fatal blood-borne disease. About 5–7% of freshly-caught lobsters bear the disease, which can spread rapidly among other lobsters concentrated in the pounds. Provided at 2.5 mg per gram of feed (the consumption by one lobster), the treatment occurs as pulses of five days several times during late August and early spring. There is a mandatory one-month withdrawal time. These are the lobsters that will be sold to consumers between Christmas and March. The industry checks regularly for tetracycline resistance, but has not yet found any. Emergence of resistance would certainly be of concern, since only oxytetracycline is currently approved for this purpose.

The times of withdrawal before marketing are dependent on the total amount of antibiotic given for treatment and the

ability of the antibiotic to remain in the fish once therapy has
been discontinued. The timing between withdrawal and sales
is based on studies looking at how long residues actually remain in the body of the fish. Ideally, antibiotic treatments of
fish are kept to short time periods, thus eliminating the
buildup of these drugs in the fish. While the concerns of the
consumer regarding antibiotic residues in the fish may be answered by these control measures, the broad ecologic effects
of antibiotic use here are the same as those elsewhere.

The Catfish Industry

About 600 million pounds of catfish are produced annually in
the United States and sold on the wholesale market (Figure
7.2, page 197). The industry, valued at over $700 million, is
centered in the southeastern United States, principally the
state of Mississippi, followed by Alabama, Arkansas, Georgia,
Florida, and Louisiana.

Catfish ponds vary greatly in terms of size and general
farming practices. Farms can be as large as 20–30 acres for the
typical commercial pond in the Mississippi Delta or as small
as one quarter of an acre on a private farm (Figure 7.2). Commonly the farmer stocks his ponds so that he will have a load
of about 5000 fish per acre. In more intensive farming with
aeration, the number of fish can reach 8,000 per acre. The
typical single-family farms may have small ponds, the so-
called "mom and pop" ponds, which contain only about 2,000
fish per acre. Harvesting in the small farms consists of
drainage of the ponds and collection of the fish left in the
residual water. This is usually done in the winter. Ponds of
large commercial enterprises generally are not drained. Most
commercial units employ nets that collect only the larger,
more mature fish and allow the smaller fish to pass through.
They then restock the ponds to achieve the optimum population. The companies add more water to make up for evapora-

tion. These different practices influence the conditions the catfish must endure, the kinds of diseases they might contract, and the ways they might contract them.

Antibiotics may enter the scene as soon as disease becomes evident. Whenever dead fish surface, the farmer has two choices. One is to take away the feed and let the fish recover on their own; the other is to add antibiotics, generally as feed additives (Figure 7.3, page 198). The latter practice is decreasing. The common bacterial diseases, namely, those of the skin or blood, are caused by gram-negative bacteria of the *Aeromonas* and *Edwardsiella* types. Fish are more susceptible to infections at temperatures between 22 and 28°C (72–82°F). Below 28°C, the immune systems of fish are not active, so they are more likely to become diseased; below 22°C bacteria do not survive well, so the fish are protected. Thus, between 22 and 28°C, higher numbers of bacteria are present in the pond and fish have depressed immune systems. Consequently, infection becomes more probable. Such conditions generally occur in the spring and fall. The most popular means of treatment are tetracycline or ormetoprim combined with sulfadimethoxine added to the feed or obtained as a premixed medicated feed. The preparation is usually in an oil base so that the antibiotic will not be lost by dissolving into the water or becoming so diluted that the concentrations lose their effectiveness. In general, the tetracycline feeding continues for 10 days with a 21-day withdrawal period. The feeding of ormetoprim and sulfadimethoxine takes place for 5 days with a withdrawal time of 3 days. Ponds that are not completely drained from prior antibiotic treatments may contain considerable amounts of active drug residue after each cycle. Thus, newly introduced fish are subjected to residual antibiotics and to antibiotic-resistant bacteria.

A common infectious microorganism, *Aeromonas hydrophila*, causes sepsis in catfish and can sometimes lead to diarrhea and sepsis in certain susceptible people who might ingest the mi-

Figure 7.2. A) *Catfish harvested from a farm in Mississippi (Angelo De-Paola, United States Food and Drug Administration, Daulphin Island, Alabama). B) A typical 14-acre catfish pond (Angelo DePaola, United States Food and Drug Administration, Daulphin Island, Alabama).*

Figure 7.3. *Workers collect dead catfish floating on the pond's surface. This occurrence may indicate the need for antibacterial therapy (Angelo DePaola, United States Food and Drug Administration, Daulphin Island, Alabama).*

croorganisms. In two states, Mississippi and Alabama, 90% of these bacteria associated with the catfish ponds tested resistant to tetracyclines and other antibiotics. As in other instances, the most important consequence of tetracycline-resistant bacteria for this industry is the inability to control infections that were once treatable with this relatively inexpensive drug. A further consequence is that these resistant microorganisms can be passed to humans through the food chain. In fact, resistant forms of these bacteria have been found on the carcasses of catfish being sold at market. This finding raises more environmental concern than medical fears, since these bacteria are not particularly infectious to people. The chances of this transfer occurring is minimal once the fish is cooked. "Pickup" of these bacteria, however, can occur on hands during preparation in the home and, thus, they can eventually reach the intestines. The other possible source would be contamination of other foods prepared on the same kitchen surface. Therefore, it is important to wash all foods to be eaten uncooked and to prepare them on surfaces separate from those being used to prepare the raw fish.

While antibiotic residues in the fish product could be a problem, this possibility is reduced by the withdrawal of the antibiotics before harvest. Another potential adverse effect is not so easily managed, that is, the selection of resistant bacteria that will propagate and could eventually spread to the consumer on the commercial product.

It is for this reason that fish farmers are moving away from the use of antibiotics and employing improved management practices so as to avoid disease and the need for antibiotics.

The catfish industry continues to expand. At the present time, it is located only in the southeastern states. It is inevitable that this profitable industry will grow in the coming years.

Of note, in the 10 years since this book was first published, the use of antibiotics in commercial fish aquaculture has diminished considerably. By one estimate, the percentage of medicated feed sales as a percentage of total feed sales for catfish dropped from nearly 2% in 1992 to about 0.5% today. Most current antibiotic usage occurs in the raising of young fish in hatcheries and considerably less is used in the final production.

If, as we hope, the trend continues, then despite the growing industry, what had been of concern in the beginning of the last decade will not occur since these producers should follow the current practice of prudent antibiotic usage through improved management.

The Salmon Industry

Salmon farming is another industry that has used considerable amounts of antibiotics, particularly tetracyclines and sulfonamides in the past. At the beginning of the last decade, an estimated 147 pounds of antibiotic were applied per acre of salmon per year. This amount has decreased and continues to decline, although actual amounts are hard to obtain. Some salmon pens are placed in natural sea waters; the antibiotics and resultant resistant strains of bacteria created by these farms will have contact with other marine life. As a result, antibiotics used for raising salmon represent another selective force for resistant strains in yet another environmental niche.

Aware of the ecological changes accompanying salmon rearing, notably the contamination of the water beds and other marine life, lobstermen and families in northern Maine in the early 1990s fought successfully against the entry into their area of a Norwegian company wanting to set up a salmon fishery. While companies contend that the antibiotics are used only when needed, it is well known that, during crowded conditions, antibiotics are required routinely for long periods of time. Since they are deposited in the water, they can be picked up easily by other marine animals. Tetracycline is not rapidly degraded in fish. Thus, it is excreted in its active state in feces and deposited on the sea floor. Here, too, it remains relatively stable, out of direct sunlight, which can degrade it. Consequently, the ecological effect of this antibacterial agent in the sea is the same as it is in land animals. The long-term selection of resistant and multiresistant bacteria in salmon and other marine life forms not only poses a barrier to the treatment of diseases in the fish themselves, but this selection also provides a means by which these resistance genes can move into the human food chain, either on the fish themselves or through other edible marine animals.

Aside from its production of catfish, the United States is not one of the world's larger aquaculture producers. It farms only about 60 million pounds of Atlantic salmon per year, and it imports annually about 300 million pounds, mainly from Canada and Chile.

The aquaculture industry in Canada is very similar to that in the United States except that another drug, florphenicol, is currently also available. The most common antibiotic (90% of all use) is oxytetracycline. Since 1998, in Canada all of the antibiotics reaching the fish are prescribed. Most are provided to small growing fish, not those ready for harvest. This latter practice allows for as many as 12 months without antibiotic treatment before the fish come to harvest.

Norway differs considerably in its use and need of antibiotics. In this country, a large percentage of drug treatments goes for parasitic, not bacterial infections. Another kind of antibiotic, specifically, oxalinic acid (a quinolone), is used in 60–80% of applications. Norway has made drastic changes in its antibiotic policy, reducing antibiotic usage down to perhaps 10% of what it was ten years ago when this book was first published. According to the most recent data from 1998, Norway used 1.9 grams of antibiotic per ton of Atlantic salmon, whereas Canada used 151 grams per ton. This amount was down from a high of 346 grams/ton in 1997 and follows the trend of continuing reduction. The Canadian goal is to reduce levels to those currently in Norway, which represent the "gold standard" sought by many countries, including the United States. To quote Dr. M. Sheppard, a Canadian veterinary consultant with the industry, "with ever increasing vaccine efficiencies, continued improvements to farming codes of practice, and natural genetic stock selection, the overall use of antibiotics in production of salmon in British Columbia has widely declined. In the years to come, that remains the goal of all parties involved."

The attention to antibiotic use in aquaculture in the U.S., Canada, Norway, and other industrialized nations far exceeds that in animals. Drastic changes in rearing practices, associated with very significant decreases in antibiotic use, have occurred over the past decade. To some extent this change has been predicated by proper use of vaccines and new management procedures. On the other hand, it is also a response to public pressure, since most of the fish are raised in natural waters with direct potential consequences to the environment. One hopes that as we begin the new millennium, this same attention will "spill over" to other countries raising fish and into the terrestrial food animals.

Antibiotic Use in Minor Species of Animals

Sheep, goats, mink, rabbits, foxes, and other animals raised in small numbers all receive antibiotics at different times in their lives. In fowl, besides the large quantities used in treating or raising chickens and turkeys, antibiotics are also given to pheasants, quail, and ducks. Among the most important antibiotics for these purposes are the tetracyclines, penicillin G, neomycin, streptomycin, and sulfur derivatives. In these animals, as in cattle and pigs, the antibiotics are used most often for growth promotion and to increase the growth efficiency of the feed. Even minks are fed antibiotics in order to increase their pelt sizes.

All preparations are usually given as an additive to the feed, generally at low levels ranging from 20 to 50 grams per ton. Since all the antibiotics are also human therapeutics, they serve as yet another source for selection of resistant bacteria that gain access to the environmental pool shared with humans. Of course, the bacterial flora of those people having direct contact with the animals and the antibiotics will receive the greatest impact. But wherever these animals or their products are sent, bacteria can travel with them, thus entering new ecological areas.

Antibiotic Use in the Home: The Family Pet

About 40% of households in the United States have dogs. In some areas, this number may be as high as 50%. Dogs also carry antibiotic-resistant bacteria, as do cats. Studies of the feces from healthy dogs found a high frequency of antibiotic-resistant bacteria and transferable resistance determinants. By one study, 65% of almost 100 dogs carried tetracycline-resistant *E. coli*, of which most were multiresistant. Since these pets were not taking antibiotics at the time, the authors suggested that the origin of these resistant bacteria might be commercial dog food or other neighboring animals on antibiotics. In this regard, the unexpected and unexplained finding of vancomycin-resistant enterococci in dog food further supports the notion that pet foods can be a source of the spread of antibiotic-resistant bacteria. Another study, taking place in Ireland, found that about 70% of the *E. coli* isolates from dogs were multiply resistant. High levels of resistance were also recorded in Australia, where 40% of the fecal samples taken from domestic dogs contained multiresistant bacteria. These studies show that already in the 1980s, dogs in diverse geographical areas were harboring relatively high levels of antibiotic-resistant *E. coli* in their fecal flora. These strains represent another environmental constituent capable of exchanging resistance genes.

Besides those for dogs and cats, for which most antibiotics are given by veterinarian prescription, a variety of antibiotics are readily available over the counter in pet stores throughout the world for smaller animal species. Birds, rodents, and fish are some of the pets for whom these antibiotics can be purchased (Figure 7.4, next page). The drugs are packaged as capsules, tablets, or, occasionally, in liquid or powder forms. Although the total amount of these antibiotics could be considered relatively small compared with that used in animals,

Figure 7.4. *Common human therapeutics are offered over the counter for the treatment of small pets, such as fish, rodents, and birds. This is a display of different antibiotic preparations for treating fish.*

humans, and agriculture, their easy availability has potentially unfavorable consequences.

The way that these antibiotics are distributed also raises some important questions and problems. Of particular note, the form and appearance of these drugs are remarkably similar to antibiotics used for treating people. Perhaps this is why some pet store owners and personnel with whom I've spoken have admitted taking these antibiotics occasionally to treat themselves. They perceive these antibiotic pet preparations to be the same as those used in human medicine, and they are available without a doctor's prescription.

For instance, each tetracycline capsule for fish contains 250 mg of tetracycline. This is exactly the same formulation sold for human consumption (Figure 7.5). The price of these over-the-counter antibiotics is generally similar to that of those sold

Figure 7.5. *Two of the popular antibiotics, tetracycline and nalidixic acid, recommended for pet owners to use for their fish.*

by prescription for human use, except that the pet preparations are usually provided in boxes of 8–10 pills. Thus, for some antibiotics, they may actually be cheaper. While scanning the numerous shelves of antibiotics recommended for pets, I was struck by the brilliant colors. Each antibiotic was encased in its own bicolored capsule, some of which resembled color combinations of the same antibiotics sold for human use. The most common antibiotics were the same ones frequently used by people, namely, penicillins, tetracyclines, and sulfonamides. Their uses, as indicated on the packages, are for treating obvious signs of disease, such as failure to eat or diarrhea.

The advice for antibiotic treatment generally comes from the pet store owner or worker in response to a query from the pet owner. Jack, the manager of one pet store I visited, explained a common scenario. "A pet owner comes in to me and describes the pet's problems—diarrhea, ruffled feathers, shortness of breath. Based on the kinds of symptoms and descriptions, I prescribe an antibiotic."

When I asked how he made his decisions, he simply answered, "based on my own experience." If the pet does not recuperate within the next two days, Jack simply prescribes a second antibiotic. Usually he begins by prescribing one of the tetracycline preparations. If that doesn't work, his second choice is erythromycin.

Jack's familiarity with the antibiotic names was surprising to me, but did not seem particularly unusual to him. I asked if he had a background in pharmacology. "None," he replied, "But I've been in the pet business for a long time."

Jack has worked in this particular store for over ten years and now manages it. All kinds of pet fish and products for fish are displayed in the more than 1,000 square feet of shelf space. There are other areas furnishing antibiotics and other treatments for birds, rodents, and other small animals. Shelves and tables all around the store display foods and medications for these pets. Jack, with unabashed aplomb, explained the use of antibiotics for the treatment of different pet fish. He saw no problem with the fact that pet owners ask him for advice, and that his initial suggestion is to start with an antibiotic. He sees his role as that of a practitioner giving out all kinds of drugs, including antibiotics. Yet, these are the same antibiotics that require a doctor's prescription when given to humans.

Jack admitted that he has used an antibiotic prepared for fish for himself. Once he had an inflamed finger that was bothering him and looked infected. So, he called his friend who is a nurse to ask for some advice. She told him that at the hospital doctors usually treat this kind of problem with erythromycin. So, according to Jack, "I knew that we had human-grade erythromycin for fish." "It's an antibiotic made under the same conditions as for humans," Jack explained.

"So, I went and took it." His finger got better. Jack said that he is not the only one who takes antibiotics meant for pets. At professional meetings he has learned that this is not an unusual practice, nor is it of any great concern to pet store owners and workers.

Jack claimed that he knows which of the antibiotics are human grade and which are not. Although all labels do state "not for human use," the shop owners know that it may be human grade. Jack is aware that those without a human-grade designation may not be as pure or sterile and might not be prepared in a way that is guaranteed harmless to people. In general, the non-human-grade products are those sold in bulk to the pet store owners to use in their resident animals and fish. These include a broad range of antibiotics: tetracycline, erythromycin, sulfur drugs, ampicillin, puromycin, and neomycin.

Our primary concern here is not that antibiotics are being used for these pets. If they are sick and antibiotics are needed, they should get them. The antibiotics sold, however, are the very ones used currently for humans. More importantly, in contrast to human preparations, these are readily available to pet owners for personal use. Treating the family pet will lead to the same kind of ecological phenomenon that occurs with antibiotic use anywhere, that is, selection of resistant bacteria. While these bacteria may not be infectious for humans, they do add to the environmental pool of resistance genes that can be transferred to bacteria of all kinds, including those associated with people. And in the case of the intestinal *E. coli*, the bacteria can become part of the owner's intestinal flora. Again, I am not advising against this use, only that it be appropriate.

You can buy eight 200 mg capsules of erythromycin for fish for less than $5.00, an excellent price by human drug standards. The same antibiotic and newer members of this antibi-

otic family are enjoying a comeback in human medicine because of their broadened effectiveness against microorganisms
causing skin and respiratory diseases. Furthermore, new for-
mulations make the antibiotic less irritable to the gastrointestinal tract. Resistance to erythromycin has emerged in
some of the bacteria for which this drug is used in humans.
We discussed the current problem surrounding erythromycin-resistant streptococcus in Finland and the association between this finding and increased sales of erythromycin
for human use in Finland. We can wonder whether or not resistance problems are emerging in bacteria that cause animal
and pet fish diseases. While it has never been shown, there is
also the possibility that resistance traits selected in fish bacteria could be transferred to bacteria associated with humans.
This scenario is not farfetched, since these kinds of transfers
can be detected among bacteria in the laboratory.

These are hypothetical events. What is of known concern is
the fact that people visiting pet shops have easy access to therapeutics presently used by humans. These include ampicillin
(a modified penicillin with broad antibacterial activity used
widely in human medicine), kanamycin (an aminoglycoside
used in treating childhood diseases), and nalidixic acid (used
in urinary tract infections and certain diarrheas). You may remember that nalidixic acid is the forefather of the fluoroquinolone family of antimicrobial agents with activity against
a wide group of bacteria causing urinary tract infections, bone
infections, and septicemias. As you learned, resistance to these
new drugs has appeared in bacteria that cause human disease.
Whenever these drugs are used for human or nonhuman purposes, resistance traits can be selected; therefore, appropriate-
ness in their applications should be the standard everywhere.

But the problem doesn't end with the easy availability of
single agents. An imported group of antibiotics prepared for
pet fish consists of preparations with a broad activity range,

that is, an effectiveness against many different kinds of bacteria. One of these products contains a combination of antibiotics. Besides the mixing of a sulfonamide and trimethoprim (which is one of the few combinations of antimicrobials used in human medicine), the same medication includes a third antibiotic, called metronidazole, a drug used in treating anaerobic infections. These latter infections are caused by bacteria in the bowel that cannot grow in air. Placing three potent antimicrobials in one medication means that one treatment will distribute three different powerful agents into the immediate environment with the potential to select resistant forms to any one or *all three*.

Another antibiotic formulation for fish has four different antibiotics provided as "flakes" that could be given to fish according to the pet owner's discretion. The decision would be made based on the apparent symptoms of the pet as summarized on the cylindrical container. The top of the container is turned, as for pepper and spices, and out come the specific flakes of antibiotic wanted. Flake A is chloramphenicol, to be used for cottonlike fluff on mouths and fins, ulcers, and other similar maladies. Flake B, tetracycline, attacks "fin and tail rot." Flake C, dihydrostreptomycin, treats weight loss, fading colors, or loss of scales, while Flake D, a combination of metronidazole, sulfadimethoxine, and trimethoprim, is suggested for "introducing new fish," "swollen body," or "swimming on the side."

All these descriptions are expected to be understood easily by the pet fish owner. These antibiotics have very special uses in human medicine and are rarely, if ever, found together. The kind of decision-making process used in selecting a treatment for fish and other pets may not differ greatly from the kinds of decisions that people are moved to make when seeking medical treatment or when treating themselves. This product labeling exemplifies how real the concept of indiscriminate antibiotic ingestion is to human consumers and how it indirectly challenges the "antibiotic by prescription" rule of human medicine. The relaxed attitude toward using these antibiotics for pets is perhaps reflective of the same attitude toward the use of these drugs in people. If people can give antibiotics to their pets, which many regard almost as dearly as family, why shouldn't they treat themselves or their loved ones? Although neither the pet store industry nor the companies producing these drugs are promoting such an attitude, the real-life situation lends itself to such abuses.

In an indirect and subtle way, the respect for antibiotics that we would like to engender in people is undermined by the ready access and self-medication involved in treating household pets. While the quantity of this antibiotic use is small in the scheme of things, these applications are everyday occurrences. We must consider them seriously, at least at some level, in our efforts to preserve a concerned respect toward these irreplaceable drugs.

The examples we have discussed in this chapter further illustrate how ubiquitously antibiotics are used in every aspect of our lives. Therefore, is it any wonder that we have antibiotic resistance? Our point throughout is to be aware of the consequence of this use, since it bears on the present and future efficacy of these precious drugs.

chapter eight

Future Prospects

New Advances against Impending Disaster

The past two decades have witnessed a continued unprecedented rise in the emergence and spread of antibiotic resistance determinants among disease-causing bacteria. These resistant bacteria have colonized ecological niches in countries worldwide, making all geographic areas vulnerable to the problem of ineffective therapy for bacterial diseases. This situation raises the staggering possibility that a time will come when antibiotics as a mode of therapy will be only a fact of historic interest. While scientific advances may eventually offer a way to replace antibiotics with other means of treating disease, we would rather make that decision ourselves instead of being forced to abandon antibiotic therapies because they have become useless. Despite innovative work on vaccines and other methods of increasing our body's defenses against infection, most scientists and physicians cannot imagine a future without antibiotics.

As for the foreseeable future, I do not envision complete antibiotic failure. Most bacteria are still susceptible to at least some of the antibiotics available currently. The choice of effective antibiotics, however, is growing narrower and harder to make while new antibiotics are making their way into the marketplace very slowly. We have already reached the point where the cost and availability of particular antibiotics have compromised therapy in certain parts of the world.

Some analysts warn of present-day scenarios in which infectious antibiotic-resistant bacteria devastate whole human populations. They say, "Isn't this already the situation with resistant strains of *Staphylococcus aureus?*" These bacteria, often called "golden staph" because of the gold color of the colonies on laboratory agar, are the scourge of hospitals, where they cause surgical and blood-borne infections characterized by high fevers, sweats, and drops in blood pressure. Death is not uncommon.

In the late 1970s and early 1980s, multiresistant golden staph plagued hospitals in Melbourne, Australia. This situation certainly epitomized the gravest of antibiotic resistance problems. At first insidious and unrecognized, these multiply resistant staphylococci soon became evident as the cause of death among unsuccessfully treated patients in hospitals throughout the Melbourne area. The problem surfaced not just in one hospital but in many.

The situation raised such havoc and fear that ambulance drivers wore masks to protect themselves from "catching" the golden staph. The concern was not unjustified. Hospital microbiologists and infection control nurses traced the resistant microorganism to hospital personnel and to inanimate objects, including the hospital linens and washing facilities. While this kind of bacteria is always difficult to treat, the Melbourne strain was resistant to all traditional first-line antibiotics. It was also resistant to antiseptics, making this form of cleaning ineffective. Only one antibiotic, vancomycin, remained effective. But this drug was very expensive and also potentially toxic, and, therefore, had to be used sparingly.

The severity of the hospital staphylococcus problem in Melbourne spurred the formation of a local group of hospital personnel who sought to curb and control the spread of the microorganism. They surmised that proper hygiene, notably handwashing among doctors and nurses, and containment of infected patients in designated areas would help. Additionally, they suggested more appropriate use of antibiotics, the source of resistance selection. Out of this group effort came the development and publication of a booklet called *Antibiotic Guidelines*, which explained how to use antibiotics more wisely. Besides producing the book, the developers used innovative ways to publicize it (Figure 8.1).

This critical real-life problem formed the core example for a British BBC and American "Nova" TV documentary in 1984, which focused on the global problem of antibiotic resistance. Fortunately, by using vancomycin and initiating broad public health measures among hospital personnel and hospital services, the Melbourne hospitals were eventually able to contain the microorganism and its spread. But the problem remains prominent in hospitals there, where 20–40% of the *S. aureus* are still multiply resistant today. The Australians learned a lot from the experience. Public health measures did help control spread of these resistant bacteria. But everybody realized that antibiotic resistance could emerge as a devastating, nearly uncontrollable health problem. In this Melbourne epidemic, the "worst case" scenario was experienced.

What if this kind of event were to occur today? It is not out of the realm of possibility. Less than a decade later, vancomycin resistance emerged in the microorganisms known as enterococci, which exchange other resistance genes with staphylococci. Moreover, vancomycin resistance is not confined to one kind of determinant. There are five different re-

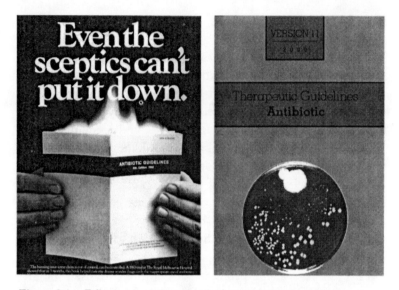

Figure 8.1. *Following a massive outbreak of multiresistant* Staphylococcus au- reus *in Melbourne hospitals in the late 1970s and early 1980s,* Antibiotic Guide- lines *was compiled and distributed as a means to improve antibiotic usage. Antibi- otic misuse was considered one of the reasons for the propagation of these resistant strains. The book was publicized in order to get its message across to practitioners. The* Guidelines *is now in its eleventh edition and used throughout Australia.*

sistance determinants that can mediate vancomycin resis- tance, four of which are transferable.

Emergence of a vancomycin-resistant MRSA was the crisis expected in the beginning of the 1990s. In fact, in 1992, Bill Noble in London reported the transfer of vancomycin resis- tance from enterococci to *Staphylococcus aureus* in his labora- tory on agar plates and even on the skin of a mouse. It is therefore surprising that such a transfer event has not yet been observed clinically. Instead, strains of staphylococci have emerged with resistance mediated through chromosomal mu- tations in the target for the drug. Fortunately, these vancomycin-resistant *Staphylococcus aureus* (VRSA) strains have not reached large proportions, but they have caused suffering, treatment failures, and death. Two new drugs that can treat this organism appeared at the end of the decade: the streptogramins (*Synercid*) and the oxazolidinones (*Zyvox*). Already in defense, strains of staphylococcus and enterococcus have emerged with resistance to these new drugs. This resistance, which has appeared in several patients, needs to be contained. Caution and prudent use of vancomycin and the newer drugs must be overriding factors so as to prevent the further emergence and propagation of these kinds of resistant bacteria. Certainly, there continues to be an increasing need for new antibiotics to treat these potentially fatal infections. Clearly, the relief from MRSA that vancomycin provided for almost 15 years is no longer guaranteed. Either through the transfer of resistance (via plasmids) or the spread of resistant staphylococci, more and more patients are at risk of contracting this difficult-to-treat infection. No one can afford to be complacent. We must all heed these potentially disastrous events when they appear and work toward preventing similar occurrences in the future as new drugs reach the clinical arena.

As we mentioned earlier, another "close call" with antibiotic failure occurred in the early 1980s in Zaire, where multiresistant *Shigella dysenteriae*, which causes severe and often bloody diarrhea, claimed hundreds of lives. These infectious bacteria were resistant to all commonly used antibiotics. Only nalidixic acid was effective, and in many cases, it was administered too late. Moreover, within a year after nalidixic acid was introduced, strains resistant to this antimicrobial appeared and thwarted treatment. In this *Shigella* epidemic, however, it was the only drug available. For some it was life-saving; for others it proved too late or altogether useless.

A recent endemic of typhoid fever occurred in Tajikistan, where almost 9,000 people were infected and 95 died. The organism, *Salmonella typhi*, was resistant to seven different antibiotics, including all the first-line agents. The clinicians did not have newer agents with which to treat this devastating health crisis. The multidrug resistance of this typhoid fever organism had evolved significantly from the chloramphenicol-resistant strains of the 1970s that caused confusion and death in Mexico and parts of Central America because of unanticipated resistance and inadequate treatment.

While these three examples may seem like unusual isolated incidents, they are not. Other smaller outbreaks of hard-to-treat, resistant infections have surfaced in different parts of the world—in the general community as well as in hospitals. Some of these we have discussed earlier—tuberculosis in New York, salmonellosis in Illinois. They offer a bleak picture for the future as such events continue to occur. There needs to be an improvement in our understanding and acknowledgment of the resistance problem in order to prevent such incidents from reaching calamitous proportions. Certain common facts and features underlying the emergence and spread of antibiotic resistance merit comment.

Resistance Can Be Reversed

As we discussed earlier, faced with rising erythromycin-resistant *Streptococcus pyogenes* (the cause of "strep throat"), concerned physicians in Finland advocated reduced usage of erythromycin through a country-wide educational campaign. Remarkably, the country's medical profession responded to the appeal. While it took time—about two years—resistance rates dropped from a high of about 20% to 8% nationwide.

In another example, the use of avoparcin as a growth promotant in animals was not foreseen as a public health problem until later, when vancomycin became the drug of choice for the treatment of patients with MRSA. Only then did the structural similarity between avoparcin and vancomycin become clear. Bacteria (initially the enterococcus) selected with resistance to avoparcin were cross-resistant to vancomycin. The intestinal flora of individuals living in countries where avoparcin was used in food production contained easily detectable levels of vancomycin-resistant enterococci. First in Denmark, then in other parts of Scandinavia, and finally throughout Europe, avoparcin was banned from livestock. What followed over the ensuing two years was a dramatic decrease in the carriage rate of vancomycin-resistant enterococci associated with the animals and animal products, and even in the intestinal tracts of people living in the countries.

As discussed above, reversal of resistance does not occur rapidly. Resistant organisms are not necessarily in a less "fit" state. They can easily survive in the environment since there is no selection against them. However, without a selective advantage, in time the resistant organisms will be replaced by susceptible ones. This is the route most feasible for reversing resistance—encourage the return of a susceptible flora. With a susceptible microbial environment, when an infection does occur, the organism will respond to the antibiotic armamentarium that we have.

Low-Level Resistance Precedes High-Level Resistance

Studies of certain respiratory and urinary tract pathogens alert us to an interesting biological phenomenon—low-level resistance precedes high-level resistance. At the International Congress of Infectious Diseases a few years ago, Dr. Fernando Baquero of the Hospital Ramon y Cajal in Madrid showed that the first penicillin-resistant strains of meningococcus, gonococcus, and even pneumococcus that appeared were only slightly less susceptible (more resistant) than the susceptible strains. In most cases, these low-level mutants were not of concern because the resistance could be over-whelmed with a high dose of antibiotic. Following closely on the heels of these low-level resistant variants, however, were those with higher resistances. What had happened was that, with time, these or other strains had picked up genes having more powerful mechanisms of resistance to these antibiotics, including those on plasmids and on transposons. Dr. Baquero proposed that we should pay more attention to these low-level resistant variants when they are seen in hospital or clinic bacteriology units because they usually herald the eventual appearance of the higher-level resistant types that truly com-promise treatment.

A similar picture has emerged with fluoroquinolone resis-tance. Bacteria need several mutations before they become fully resistant to treatment levels of fluoroquinolones. The first step, generally a mutation in the enzyme (topoisomerase) target of the fluoroquinolones, decreases susceptibility to the drug. However, these bacteria are still susceptible to the doses of fluoroquinolones generally given for treatment. But the first-step mutants are forerunners of subsequent mutant strains, which provide higher and higher levels of resistance. These organisms thwart treatment. These second, third, and fourth mutations confer further changes in the targets of the drug. In addition, they cause increased expression of a protein pump, which exports the fluoroquinolones out of the cell so they cannot do damage inside the cell.

The appearance of vancomycin-resistant *Staphylococcus au-reus* (VRSA) also occurs through multiple chromosomal mu-tation steps. There are reports, for instance, of methicillin-resistant *Staphylococcus aureus* strains in which a minority of the population of bacteria (one in a million to one in a ten million) appear insensitive to vancomycin. Called "heteroge-neously" resistant to vancomycin, these strains were initially considered a clinical curiosity. But, in fact, in a number of studies these mutants have led to treatment failure. In one group of orthopedic patients, twelve out of fourteen patients failed treatment with vancomycin because the MRSA strains were heterogeneously resistant to the drug. The orthopedic prostheses had to be removed. In these cases the resistance problem did not involve immunocompromised patients, but otherwise healthy surgical patients. These kinds of mutants are precursors to the more fully vancomycin-resistant strains that result from further mutations.

In most resistant bacteria the mutational progression to resistance is very different from what happens when bacteria acquire resistance genes on transposons and plasmids. Here, the level of antibiotic resistance expressed is far higher than what is actually needed to resist a therapeutic dose of antibiotics. The resistance determinants are providing an excess of resistance power. It is like taking a mallet to kill a fly. This finding suggests that the evolution of resistance determinants was probably not merely a response to accommodate the antibiotic levels that we use. Perhaps it was not even for the purpose of fighting antibiotics. These determinants may actually have another function in nature that eludes scientific investigators. In any case, they become more frequent when they are selected by the antibiotics to which they render their bacterial hosts resistant.

One Antibiotic Can Select for
Resistance to Others

There is another feature of resistance that adds to the problem—"linkage" of resistance genes. Since most plasmids and even many transposons contain genes for resistance to different antibiotics, the use of any one of these antibiotics will select bacteria with resistance to all of them. This event will occur immediately if the multiresistant bacteria are already there. But, even if they are not initially evident, they can be recruited, as we discussed before, by chronic use of a single antibiotic. The appearance of multidrug resistance in the intestinal bacteria of animals and farm dwellers followed prolonged oxytetracycline use in animal feeds. Likewise, multidrug resistance eventually appeared in people taking a single antibiotic for acne or urinary tract infection. While initially the drug selects bacteria resistant to itself, with time multiple resistance emerges from genes acquired elsewhere. And, as noted earlier, tetracycline or chloramphenicol can select *Escherichia coli* mutants that are resistant via a chromosome mutation not only to the antibiotic doing the selection but also to others *unrelated* to it. Among the resistances so selected is low-level resistance to the quinolones. If the use of one antibiotic can indirectly select mutants to others, we can see that the resistance problem, in all its complexity, poses an immense challenge to the future.

New Drugs May Be Subject to the Activity of Old Resistance Determinants

A setback to new discovery is the relatively recent observation that resistance to the newer drugs is appearing faster than ever expected. Within less than a decade, resistances have compromised use of the newer cephalosporins, penicillins, trimethoprim, and trimethoprim-sulfamethoxazole combinations, the new aminoglycosides and the fluoroquinolones.

New drugs, introduced into the clinical arena, may run into a resistance "roadblock" within as short a period as two years. Why? Part of the answer relates to their heavy usage and the selection of resistance as with other drugs. Mass marketing takes place in order to sell enough of the new drug to make up for the large expense of developing it. A new drug becomes a "fad," something physicians (and their patients) want to use. Thus, large amounts of the drug are presented to the bacterial ecosystem—just the right selective force for propagating the rare mutants bearing resistance mechanisms for that drug.

Another part of the problem is the lack of structural uniqueness in these new drugs. Generally, newly discovered drugs are tested and designed to be invulnerable to the known resistance determinants. If a new drug, however, is structurally related to an older one, the new antibiotic may eventually be inactivated by the same old resistance mechanisms. Under heavy use, the drug may select for rare mutant forms of these "old" resistance determinants—mutant proteins that can now inactivate the newer form of the antibiotic (Figure 8.2). This possibility was vividly brought home in the emergence of resistances to the newest penicillins and cephalosporins. In Germany, a plasmid encoding resistance to the new cephalosporins appeared in a clinical strain of *Klebsiella*, a potential cause of pneumonias and systemic infections. A genetic study showed that the gene for the enzyme that degraded the antibiotic was the same as one that destroyed the simpler, older cephalosporins. A couple of mutations in the gene for the enzyme had occurred that extended the structural forms of cephalosporins that the enzyme could destroy.

The best reconstruction of events leading to this new determinant would be that random mutations occurred during the many duplications of the old resistance gene. In most cases these mutations would be inconsequential and would be diluted out by all the normal genes. One of these mutations, however, allowed the bacteria to survive in the presence of the new cephalosporin antibiotic. These bacteria propagated under the antibiotic selection. Once the new gene became a significant part of the environmental pool of resistance, it could be transferred to other bacteria and the persistence of the new resistance determinant would be assured.

Another example comes from a number of outbreaks in different countries of resistant intestinal bacteria capable of destroying the newer generation of penicillins. Again, genetic analysis showed these genes to be mutations of the very common TEM-1 ß-lactamase gene—the gene that specifies an en-

222

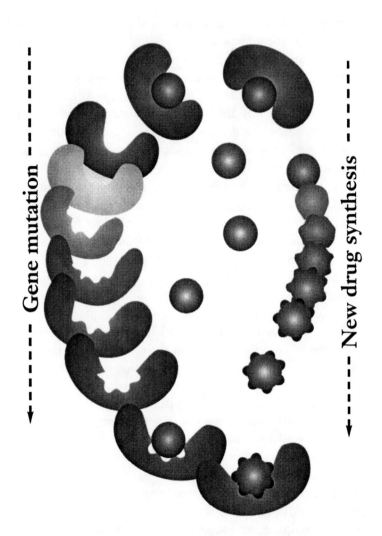

Figure 8.2. *Bacteria have acquired resistance genes for ß-lactamases, which are able to break down newer forms of penicillins and cephalosporins. ß-lactamases with an increased spectrum of activity result from small mutations in a previous ß-lactamase gene with a narrower spectrum of activity. The new mutant protein now accommodates and destroys the newer ß-lactam antibiotics (Bonnie Marshall, Tufts University School of Medicine).*

zyme that breaks the ß-lactam ring of penicillins and so inactivates the antibiotic. Natural mutations, at rates of one in a million to one in 100 million, had led to a form of the enzyme that could detoxify all of these new drugs. Like the cephalosporin-degrading enzymes, these "new" penicillin-destructive enzymes have become increasingly evident.

These ß-lactamase changes are examples of how evolution (in this case, that of a single gene), combined with strong antibiotic selection, can forge new resistances from old resistance determinants. Today, almost 90 different TEM–1-like ß-lactamases have emerged. Members of this new family of resistance enzymes can destroy the old penicillins as well as any of the new penicillin derivatives currently on the market. This will probably extend to others making their way into clinical practice. Thus, they threaten the therapeutic use and efficacy of these newer antibiotics.

New Drugs and New Approaches Are Needed

To address and deal with the present resistance problems, investigators in drug research have immersed themselves in the task of discovering and developing new antibiotics that are not subject to known antibiotic resistance mechanisms. If a drug is totally new, resistance mechanisms may not yet have been selected. But such truly "new" antibiotics are harder and harder to find. Researchers seeking new antibiotics among bacteria and fungi in soils often end up discovering the same kinds of antibiotics that have been found before, or subtle variations of them. If the drug does not differ greatly from prior antibiotics, it will be thwarted by resistance mechanisms already in existence.

The leaders of recent drug discovery programs are now casting their nets elsewhere to find new antibiotics. One potential source is in the new kinds of bacteria recovered from drilling miles beneath the earth's surface. Another innovative source is insects from which antibiotic-like substances have been discovered recently. Meanwhile, other investigators have identified antibacterial compounds in the skin of frogs. Michael Zasloff was led to discover these substances by observing that frogs did not become infected after surgery and placement back into water in which bacteria were prominent. Extracts of the skin provided the answer—antibiotic substances that he named "magainins." Curiously, other scientists found new antibiotics in our own white cells, the neutrophils, that circulate in our blood. These substances have been called "defensins" since they act to defend the body against bacteria, viruses, and fungi.

These new types of "antibiotics," such as magainins and defensins, form the core of a larger family of "peptide" antibiotics. They offer some optimism because they differ strikingly from those currently in use. The goal is to produce these new antibiotic substances in large enough quantities to be used therapeutically against infection. Since they are made of protein, however, there is concern that they may be recognized by the body as foreign and removed by antibodies of the person's immune system. Moreover, as with other antibiotics, these new ones risk succumbing to the same ecological fate— the selection of mutants resistant to them. The likelihood and time frame for the appearance of such mutants will depend not only on the nature of the antibiotic itself but also on how much and how often it is used. It is not surprising that the more a killing agent is used, the more likely it is to select a rare mutant that can resist it. Still, the finding of truly new agents is an important advance.

A more recent approach to discovering new antibiotics evolves from advancements in DNA sequencing, namely, deciphering the genetic sequence of total bacterial chromosomes. By comparing chromosomal genes from different disease-causing bacteria, investigators can find new potential targets for new antibiotics. By comparisons with the human genome, targets can be selected that do not appear in human cells. From these novel targets will come new chemical entities—our new antibiotics—that attack bacteria but leave the patient unharmed. This approach shows promise, but no new drugs have yet emerged from this work. The path from target identification to discovering which natural or synthetic products will inhibit these targets can be long. On the other hand, we should regard these efforts optimistically, since they imply that companies are willing to invest in long-term efforts, even for decades, before the introduction of new antibiotics. At the same time, our prime objective should be the prudent use of all current and newly created antibiotics so as to preserve their efficacy for future generations.

Other findings also support optimism. Some resistant bacterial strains may be able to accommodate one kind of resistance, but not others. More specifically, resistance to some antibiotics may increase the bacterium's susceptibility to others. But which ones are they? Shouldn't we find out? Perhaps once bacteria become resistant to one drug they become more sensitive to another. Evidence for this kind of phenomenon has come from studies of tetracycline resistance. Bacteria resistant to tetracycline by means of a membrane protein that pumps tetracycline out of the cell are more susceptible to aminoglycoside antibiotics, such as kanamycin and gentamicin. These kinds of antibiotics are used clinically with caution within very defined maximal levels because of their inherent toxicity to the kidney. If less of these antibiotics could be used, the side effects would be greatly reduced and their efficacy would be improved.

In a still more unexpected example, salicylates, the ingredient in aspirin, can cause some bacteria to increase resistance to certain antibiotics but at the same time gain sensitivity to others. We could profit from devoting energy toward looking at the consequences to the host bacterium of bearing resistance to an antibiotic. While the resistance mechanism may be helpful in the face of the antibiotic, it may be a detriment to other functions of the bacteria. The resistance may reduce the bacterium's ability to cause disease by causing changes in its cell wall. For example, research scientists noted that some pneumococci that became more resistant to penicillin via cell wall changes were less able to produce disease. A microorganism called *Bordetella*, which causes whooping cough, has resistance and virulence genes intricately linked. Mutations in one or more genes have the potential to create negative consequences on others in this bacterium. Some of these negative effects may be subtle and are presently unknown. If discovered, they could be used to an advantage. For instance, knowing that bacteria bearing a resistance trait can no longer live at a particular temperature or in a particular acidic or basic environment could allow us to develop alternative ways to destroy them. In other words, treatment can be aimed directly at those bacteria bearing a particular resistance determinant.

A different research approach has attempted to produce drugs that will cure bacteria of their resistance elements. For instance, certain chemicals inhibit the multiplication of plasmids. If the plasmid is not duplicated, each new daughter cell will theoretically be free of the plasmid and its linked resistances. But this approach is up against a major stumbling block. While many of these resistance determinants lie on extrachromosomal DNA elements, such as plasmids, they also reside on chromosomes in the form of transposons. Therefore, the curing of a plasmid will never assure removal of the determinant. Since it lies on a transposon, it can be transferred onto another chromosome, where it will remain stable. If we go after the chromosome, we are essentially doing what antibiotics do—killing the bacterial cell.

Natural selection has already complicated this approach. Genetic studies by Ron Skurray and his research team in Melbourne, Australia, showed how resistance genes, formerly on plasmids, have moved onto chromosomes of resistant staphylococci. This movement to the chromosomes has had two major effects, one for the determinant and the other for the cell. When the resistance gene is on the chromosome, it is more stable. It is no longer susceptible to the vagaries of a plasmid that can be lost spontaneously by the cell. By moving onto the chromosome, the determinant and the cell no longer need the plasmid. The cell, in losing its resistance plasmids, can then accommodate other plasmids more easily—namely, those bearing new resistances. Thus, like a new book in a library, a new resistance gene first enters the cell and circulates freely on the plasmid. With time, it is put out of rapid circulation into the chromosome, the cell's "permanent non-circulating collection" (Figure 8.3, next page).

There is, of course, the possibility of designing a compound that would specifically interfere with the replication of transposons. One way is to introduce genetic material that interrupts the duplication and/or spread of the transposon. If transposons could be eliminated, such treatments could selectively remove a multitude of resistance determinants from their natural reservoirs, whether they be on chromosomes or plasmids. Because the approach deals with transposons and not the entire bacterial cell, it would maintain the natural ecology of the normally harmless bacterial host strains, such as the skin and intestinal flora. It would not lead to a change in the normal flora. Instead of killing, it would act by selectively removing the "passenger" resistance genes. The approach would maintain this important normal skin and intestinal flora, which protect us from invasion by more harmful varieties. If cured of their transferable resistances, these bacteria would no longer pose the threat of transferring resistance to more harmful bacteria that might enter these areas.

Some new drugs are currently in clinical studies: daptomycin, a structurally new antibiotic (from Cubist Pharmaceuticals); a vancomycin derivative (from Eli Lilly and Company); and telithromycin (from Aventis Pharmaceuticals), a member

Figure 8.3. *In* Staphylococcus aureus, *resistance genes (A,B,C) enter on plasmids that multiply. Later in time, the genes find a place on the chromosome. This event allows other plasmids of similar types to enter with different resistance genes. This phenomenon has led to the recruitment of multiple genes for resistance in a single* S. aureus *strain (Bonnie Marshall, Tufts University School of Medicine).*

of a new class of agents called ketolides. All treat gram-positive organisms, especially problem organisms like MRSA and VRE. A glycylcycline, a derivative of tetracycline (from American Home Products), is a broad-spectrum drug undergoing clinical trials. It shows good activity against tetracycline and multidrug-resistant gram-positive and gram-negative bacteria.

Rational Design of New Drugs

Scientists and clinicians must stay ahead in this struggle with microbes both by discovering new antibiotics and by uncovering novel ways to combat resistance. They must find a way to make the best use of the antibiotics now available, while seeking alternative approaches and new drugs. One approach has been to introduce chemical changes into members of the present array of antibiotics so that they are no longer modifiable by the enzymes associated with resistance. The historic example is methicillin, developed to resist penicillin-degrading enzymes.

A more recent example is the family of fluoroquinolones that are totally synthetic. They take their core structure from the first member of the quinolone group, nalidixic acid, the drug used in the *Shigella* epidemic in Zaire. As mentioned previously, this synthetic group, discovered in the 1960s, lost favor because bacteria became spontaneously resistant to it at a frequency of about one in ten million. This mutation rate is too high when hundreds of millions of bacteria could be involved. In contrast, the fluoroquinolones do not select for resistance at anywhere near that frequency—more like one in 1 billion to one in 100 billion—a frequency much less apt to occur during therapy. Another seemingly protective feature of those fluoroquinolone-resistant mutants that have emerged is that the resistance determinants are found on the chromosome. Here the resistance determinant has less chance of moving to other bacteria—not the case for those resistance genes that can be transferred on transposons or plasmids. Still, as discussed earlier, over the past decade, fluoroquinolone-resistant strains of gram-positive and gram-negative bacteria have emerged by multiple mutational steps, subsequent to increased and broader use of these drugs in communities and hospitals worldwide.

Another avenue for assaulting resistance is to design decoy molecules to fool the resistance mechanism. In one example, the penicillin-degrading enzyme "zeroes in" on something that looks like penicillin. It hooks onto it and busily tries to destroy the false target while penicillin sneaks in unscathed to kill the cell.

The combination of a ß-lactamase inhibitor and a penicillin was championed by the British company Beecham Pharmaceuticals in the 1980s. Discovering clavulanate, which inhibited the degradative enzyme penicillinase, the company recognized and pursued the possibility of using it in conjunction with amoxicillin to produce a revitalized penicillin in the drug *Augmentin*. In fact, the company paved a new route to antibiotic discovery by showing the regulatory agencies that the combination drug—amoxicillin and clavulanate—was more effective than either drug alone. This one product has revealed how companies and researchers can reach a solution to resistance—identify the mechanism and design around it or block it. *Augmentin* was followed by other inhibitor/penicillin combinations, including Pfizer's *Unisyn* (sulbactam and ampicillin) and American Home Products's *Zosyn* (tazobactam and piperacillin).

A similar approach has been taken by a biopharmaceutical company, Paratek Pharmaceuticals, Inc., in Boston. The company produces new tetracyclines that are insensitive to tetracycline resistance mechanisms. The company's chemists have designed tetracycline derivatives that either block or circumvent the two known resistance mechanisms discussed earlier, active efflux and ribosomal protection. Following ongoing tests of effectiveness in animals, these new products will eventually undergo human trials.

In this kind of discovery effort, companies begin by identifying the resistance mechanisms and designing drugs to inhibit them. They do not need to look for a new target. In a sense, bacteria have "shown us their cards" so we can design strategies and new chemicals around them. It's a rational way to win the "game." Similar kinds of false substrates can be designed to attack other resistance mechanisms, such as those that involve other enzymes that modify and inactivate antibiotics, or other membrane proteins that actively export the antibiotic out of the cell.

From Discovery to Application Is
Time-Consuming and Expensive

The optimists believe that the vista for drug discoveries is limitless and that we will continue to find new antibiotics to deal with resistance problems. The pessimists say, "Let's be practical. The money needed to find these new drugs and the time required to put them into use are very long and very costly." With each new drug there is a chance of high toxicity. In fact, the vast majority of drugs never reach clinical use because of their toxic side effects when ingested or injected. The discovery and development process is a lengthy one, which could prevent the entry of new drugs into the market fast enough to keep up with the mounting problem of resistance. It usually takes over ten years for a new drug to leave the development stage and move into clinical practice. Only about 4–5% of new medicines ever make it into use. To get final approval from the U.S. Food and Drug Administration and similar agencies worldwide, companies must perform scores of time-consuming studies and complete reams of paperwork. Hundreds of millions of dollars must be spent for all the studies needed before the drug actually reaches the marketplace. Besides demonstrating that the new antibiotic can kill certain bacteria, these drugs must be tested in animals to show that they cause no harm; only then are they tested in humans, both for efficacy and toxicity. If it can pass the human "trials," the new drug finally makes it into the marketplace. Given these enormous constraints, even if one were to design an ideal drug today to deal with current antibiotic resistance problems, the drug would not be available for another decade. By then there is no guarantee it would still be effective.

One patient questioning his doctor's prescription asked, "Won't these drugs become useless if we use them too much?" His doctor replied, "There is no need to worry. We have so many antibiotics available and new ones are being discovered all the time." While this opinion may have had some validity during the heyday of antibiotic discovery, it is certainly not true now—new antibiotics are coming into the clinical arena very slowly.

A World with No Antibiotic Controls

It is somewhat fanciful to wonder, but perhaps worth considering, what would happen if there were no controls on antibiotic use and all people were freely able to use antibiotics at

their own whims. Susceptible strains would be totally eliminated and resistant ones would dominate. Would the resistant
bacteria survive? It appears that they would. There is very little evidence to suggest that resistant bacteria are less able to
compete in an ecosystem than their susceptible siblings. In
this imaginary situation, the levels of resistant bacteria would
be so high that use of any antibiotic would not be effective.

The place where the antibiotic-resistant strain has
emerged—a hospital, community, or country—would be a site
for containment of spread, *if* this location could be quaran-
tined. Unfortunately, in most cases, this would be difficult to
achieve. Imagine that a country, let's say in Southeast Asia, is
struggling with high numbers of multiple antibiotic-resistant,
disease-causing bacteria that in most people cannot be eliminated by any antibiotic. Some people in the environment
could become inadvertent "carriers" of these bacteria, since
not all people would get disease from them. This situation
would lead to the movement of these strains into new communities, and potentially anywhere else in the world. Such was
the case of a typhoid fever bacillus resistant to ampicillin, the
best antibiotic then used to treat this disease, which appeared
in patients in Los Angeles in the mid-1970s. It was later traced
to Mexico, where these patients had been visiting. As noted
earlier, public health officials have been able to identify brothels in Southeast Asia as the initial source of penicillin-resistant
bacteria causing gonorrhea, which are now found in virtually
every country of the world. Multidrug-resistant pneumococci
in France, Iceland, the United States, and elsewhere have been
traced back to Spain, where they initially emerged under heavy
antibiotic selection.

If we imagined an earth totally bathed in antibiotics, the
only bacteria surviving would be those resistant to these
drugs. The end result would be a reestablished microbial
world carrying on its usual activity, except that all members of

this microbial population, both helpful and harmful, would be untouched by the very antibiotics to which their less fortunate ancestors had succumbed. For this new "breed" of bacteria, antibiotics would be ineffective, merely a part of their environment. Antibiotics would fit into the category of environmental toxins with which bacteria would be interacting without harm during everyday activity. In fact, this is exactly how *Escherichia coli* already cope with many of the toxic elements in our gastrointestinal tract—the *E. coli* outer wall coat and efflux pumps keep out toxic chemicals, such as bile salts.

As we discussed earlier, certain bacteria have emerged with resistance to one or more antibiotics as a common characteristic. More than 90% of the species of *Proteus mirabilis* are now tetracycline resistant. In an analogous situation, more than 90% of *Staphylococcus aureus* resist penicillin, making penicillin ineffective against the vast majority of this species. In some hospitals, multidrug-resistant *Staphylococcus aureus* represent 60% of the total *Staphylococcus aureus* causing infections. Given what we are seeing already, it is not difficult to envision a total microbial change in favor of resistant forms. Under these circumstances, unless people developed a solid immunity to bacteria, we would face a dreaded time when our ability to treat infections would be doomed to failure. The world might seem like a replay of the uncontrollable plagues of the Dark Ages.

To some extent, this scenario has already come to pass in developing countries among the indigent populations. In these areas, death is a preponderant part of life. Poor sanitation leads to spread of infectious agents while antibiotic misuse propagates resistant strains. To make matters worse, these are the very countries where money is so scarce that the government cannot afford to buy the currently useful but expensive antibiotics. People are dying from diseases that were previously treatable. Can a similar situation ever threaten the affluent, developed world?

Under the present circumstances, we can extend our imagination to a situation where multiresistant microorganisms would become so dominant and of such concern that individuals would have to be checked and decontaminated microbiologically before they passed between countries. Years ago I considered such a scene to be ridiculous and totally farfetched. Today, at a time when China and the United States are asking that applicants for certain visas announce whether or not they have been infected by the AIDS virus, and other countries may demand that visitors show evidence of a recent AIDS antibody test, such ideas join the realm of possibility. Remember the plague scare in the 1990s in India, where people were examined at the airport because of concern that the organism would move from India to other parts of the world.

Imagine you are returning from a country where it is known that infectious agents with multiple resistances dwell. Examples could be *Staphylococcus aureus* or *Salmonella typhi* resistant to all available antibiotics. You might be asked to enter an isolation room, take a shower, or be otherwise sanitized before you were finally released (Figure 8.4). Many would look back fondly on the good days long gone when all you had to do was wait in line to fill out an immigration card and get your passport stamped. Trips would be lengthened not only by security checks at departure but by a new kind of security check upon arrival.

A paradigm of this situation does exist in Perth, Australia. In order to safeguard their hospitals from multiply resistant *Staphylococcus aureus*, medical personnel place all new patients entering any hospital in Perth into an isolation area first. There the patient is tested for the presence of the methicillin-resistant *Staphylococcus aureus* (MRSA). Those new patients who are not colonized by MRSA can be moved to the normal hospital wards. If MRSA are found on a patient, however, this person is placed in a ward with other patients colonized with this potentially dangerous and easily spread microorganism. Various means are used to eradicate the microorganism.

Figure 8.4.   Will we ever reach a time when entering a country requires more than passport control? (Herbert Hächler, University of Zurich, Zurich, Switzerland.)

Nonetheless, if the patient has an indwelling catheter or other foreign object in place, no treatment can eliminate all of the microorganisms that find hiding places in and on these objects. In such instances, the patient must stay in these designated MRSA areas throughout the hospitalization.

By this single measure of isolating patients with MRSA, the hospitals in Perth have kept MRSA under control and the frequency of these strains is now among the lowest in the world. This draconian measure to control the early spread of bacteria has worked, but not without psychological consequences for the patients involved. Still, the success of this practice has led to its being suggested as a means to control the early spread of resistant bacteria. It is certainly one proven avenue for controlling the entry of resistant strains into a new area, such as other hospital wards.

In the United States and other countries, a similar isolation procedure places patients with methicillin-resistant *S. aureus* or vancomycin-resistant enterococci into separate hospital rooms. Hospital staff and visitors must put on gowns and gloves before entering the room. The goal, as in Australia, is to prevent the spread of these organisms from patient to patient. How to effectively prevent spread from larger affected areas, such as whole regions or countries, to other areas is much harder to envision.

How Do We Protect the Future from Resistance?

We, in all segments of society, must try to adhere to certain principles to safeguard our future and those of future generations. Let us outline certain goals that will help us achieve a brighter outcome.

1. Consumers should use antibiotics only when needed, at the correct dosage, and for the prescribed time period.
2. Parents, students, and teachers should urge and encourage handwashing in daycare centers, schools, and homes to prevent the local spread of infectious disease agents. Reduced infection will lead to reduced antibiotic usage.
3. Public health authorities should improve public sanitation, especially water quality, in developing areas of the world where the spread of infectious diseases is high and where antibiotics are clearly needed.
4. Medical associations and schools should provide continued and updated education on current antibiotic uses to prescribers and users. This aim can be accomplished by including these subjects for discussion and presentation at medical meetings and as up-to-date

lectures to medical, dental, veterinary, and agricultural students.

5. Research scientists and drug manufacturers should continue to acquire insights into the mechanisms of resistance and the factors associated with their spread. With this information, investigators can begin to design ways to circumvent these resistances and to prevent their spread. One approach is to design antibiotic substrates that block, trick, and confound the resistance mechanisms.

6. Pharmaceutical companies should be encouraged, even by tax and patent advantages, to discover new antibiotics for which resistance mechanisms have not yet emerged and to monitor resistance in relation to marketing of the antibiotic so as to preserve its long-term efficacy.

7. Medical personnel should develop alternatives to antibiotics to treat infectious diseases. Vaccines against common bacterial diseases and improved public health measures worldwide will do much to decrease reliance on, and overuse of, antibiotics.

8. Surveillance of resistance in clinical isolates should be instituted or performed on a regular basis. This information helps epidemiologists identify areas of endemic resistance and aids doctors in the selection of appropriate antibiotics. Together they can limit spread to nonendemic areas.

The phenomenon of antibiotic resistance, including the genetics, resistance mechanisms, and their rampant spread, must be fully understood in order to protect the world population from what could become a plague of resistance. Scientists are fervently taking steps to procure this knowledge. The obstacles, however, still challenge the most determined individuals.

Part of the responsibility for appropriate antibiotic use certainly rests on all of us. The consequences of misuse affect us, our families, and our communities. The truly unsettling feature of misuse is the selection of resistant bacterial strains. They will inflict harm not only on the present-day population but also on generations to follow and potentially on a worldwide basis. We must curtail the creation of new resistant strains that, once selected, join the microbial population at large. Moreover, we must contain them once they are recognized. Above all, we must set our goals to limit practices that select and propagate antibiotic resistance, such as demanding and stockpiling these drugs.

On a more optimistic note, many individuals, local groups, and health management organizations today have initiated programs to increase awareness of antibiotic resistance and reduce consumer misuse of antibiotics. In one successful example, the Antibiotic Resistance Collaborative, a group of health agencies in Minnesota, provided to patients who presented to their physicians with cold symptoms a brightly colored "Minnesota Cough and Cold Care" kit. Directed at fulfilling the "need to be treated" factor inherent in a doctor's office visit, the kit contained over-the-counter medications for pain and nasal congestion as well as tea bags and a packet of chicken soup. The kits were a huge success. Said one individual, "when you get to take something with you, you start to feel better." This effort points out the importance of empathizing with the patients—that their symptoms are real and not "just a cold." Moreover, patients that take time off from work to see a physician usually seek something more tangible than advice. The initiative also underscores the importance of approaching consumers, as well as providers, in controlling and reversing the antibiotic resistance problem.

chapter nine

The Individual and Antibiotic Resistance

The problem with medicating yourself is that you don't know what you're doing.   **—Anonymous**

An antibiotic-resistant infection is no longer an unexpected or curious phenomenon for community physicians to observe in their patients. People of all ages and with various illnesses are becoming aware that antibiotics are no longer all-powerful. More and more parents of young children suffering from ear infections are finding that the prior successes of the penicillin drugs in treating this illness may not be repeated. They must now rely on other more costly drugs, to which they may have a toxic reaction.

Major new advances in curing cancer have been thwarted and undermined by the emergence of bacterial infections that fail to respond to old and new antibiotics alike. Thus, although the cancer may have been controlled or even cured, some 25–30% of patients may die from infectious agents, of which half may be caused by bacteria resistant to current antibiotic therapy.

Patients admitted to the hospital for organ transplants may find their course of treatment compromised by unrelenting infections that would have responded previously to effective and safe antibiotics. A person taking an antibiotic for one infection may contract another infection, this time a resistant one, through contamination of food products or through "pick up" from other people or animals in the environment. In sum, resistant forms of bacteria are all around us. We must learn to cope with them and to develop ways of reducing their numbers.

Because of the power by which antibiotics select for resistant bacteria, every person taking an antibiotic potentially contributes a bit to the environmental pool of resistant bacteria. Some do so more than others. We are, therefore, not innocent victims of the antibiotic resistance phenomenon. Moreover, each person taking an antibiotic *inappropriately* plays a larger role in the resistance problem since this is an *unnecessary* selection of antibiotic resistance. From some public health estimates, this inappropriate use may occur as much as half of all antibiotic consumption.

Many people believe that hospitals are havens for resistant bacteria. They are not necessarily wrong; however, common sources of resistant hospital strains are the newly admitted patients themselves. More specifically, they or their bacterial flora are the barometers of antibiotic use in the community, namely, the frequency of antibiotic resistance found there.

It may be disturbing to learn that any use of an antibiotic, whether appropriate or not, will do its own share of selecting resistant forms of bacteria. It would be absurd to jump from this fact to a judgment that antibiotics should, therefore, not be used. We must accept some resistance as a natural consequence of use. But "some" level of resistance is potentially controllable. It need not be widespread, nor does it have to be multiple, that is, to more than one antibiotic. Our principal goal is to improve antibiotic use so as to maintain efficacy at the same time that we whittle away at resistance. Appropriate use of antibiotics can eliminate the causative infectious bacteria without major consequences to the other bacteria in the environment. Advances in knowledge are evolving to help us. For one thing, as we have discussed before, short-term use has fewer ecologic effects, in terms of selecting multiresistant bacteria, than does chronic use for weeks at a time. In the right setting, for certain urinary tract infections, a single day's treatment is enough to cure the infection. In this instance, the antibiotic chosen needs to be one that is heavily concentrated in the urine. Its effectiveness is assured by drinking lots of fluids and repeated voiding of the bacteria in the urine. The major effect of the antibiotic is to inhibit the bacterium's ability to cling to the wall of the bladder.

On the other hand, too short a treatment, such as for pneumonia or a bone infection, would allow infectious bacteria to survive and reinfect, with potentially decreased susceptibility to the antibiotic treatment. For example, incomplete treatment is one of the presumed causes of the multidrug-resistant tuberculosis facing the world today. Therefore, an understanding of the dynamics of antibiotic activity and antibiotic selection of resistance can help lead us to use these valuable drugs successfully, safely, *and* prudently.

The world population has used antibiotics for over 50 years. The enthusiasm following the success of the sulfonamides in the 1930s was heightened by the discovery of penicillin's effectiveness in the 1940s. These events are within the current memory of many people living now. The idea that there is such an entity as a "miracle drug" that will cure all ailments lingers on, even among prescribers. The editors of the French medical journal *La Revue Prescrire*, which aims to improve standards of medical prescription in France, illustrated this fact vividly in an experiment some years ago.[1] In an example of advertising power and reader gullibility, the journal, on

April Fool's Day, advertised a pill *Panaceum* that, with one dosage, would control mental illness for a year. Unexpectedly, within days of its publication, pharmacies in France were bombarded with inquiries and orders from willing believers who were all too ready to prescribe, as well as to swallow, such a "magic" pill. Gilles Bardelay, the editor of *La Revue Prescrire*, had to go on public television to explain the joke—one he thought would have been perfectly obvious (Figure 9.1).

Individual Accessibility and Use of Antibiotics

To many individuals, the word "antibiotic," not just penicillin, still means a drug that will cure diseases of all kinds. They do not distinguish between bacterial causes and other causes of illness. This belief is, as we have mentioned repeatedly, completely false. For instance, the average person will seek an antibiotic for relief of flu symptoms, caused by a virus. As we have noted, if an antibiotic is obtainable without prescription, as in many countries in Central and South America and in Asia, the patient can buy it directly over the counter at the local pharmacy.

In most industrialized countries such as the United States, antibiotics for human consumption are available only by prescription. This practice is dictated by law because this group of drugs can have certain toxic side effects, including allergies, for which care by a physician is necessary. It is even possible to die from some of these reactions. Some of the drugs can be given only intravenously and, therefore, the patient needs expert medical facilities, usually a hospital. Finally, control over prescription drugs may have been envisioned to avoid indiscriminate use and subsequent selection of resistant forms of bacteria. The effectiveness of this safeguard is now in question.

We may ask how much of the antibiotics used in the United States comes through physicians' prescriptions and how much derives otherwise. Perhaps not surprisingly, there is a major

LES NOUVEAUX PRODUITS

PANACEUM	psychotropine (DSM 4)	
psychotrope polyvalent	Boîte de 1 comprimé à 5 mg 72.25 F	Bravo
	Séc. Soc. 70 % et coll.	
	Lab Clin-Roussel-Poulenc	

» Traitement des affections psychologiques et psychiatriques résistant aux therapeutiques usuelles ». C'est ainsi que l A M M definit sagement l'indication de ce nouveau medicament dont nous avions deja eu l'occasion de vous vanter les merites il y a quelques mois.
En realite, meme les affections non resistantes sont sensibles a Panaceum® mais on pourrait, a juste titre , craindre un effondrement des ventes des autres psychotropes qui rendent pourtant des services notables.

Figure 9.1. *The April 1984 issue of the French medical journal* La Revue Prescrire *came out on April Fool's Day. It advertised a new psychotropic drug called* Panaceum *that could control mental illness for a year. While it was intended as a joke, the overwhelming response from physicians and pharmacies wanting to know where and how to get this drug required the editor of the magazine to make a public disclaimer* (La Revue Prescrire, *Paris, France*).

proportion of the latter. For example, one investigation into the problem of antibiotic-resistant gonorrhea in a Baltimore venereal disease clinic found that 10% of patients had already taken antibiotics during the two weeks before they attended the clinic. Seventy percent of these patients took the antibiotics because they suspected they "might" have a venereal disease; the other 30% took antibiotics for other reasons. When tested, only 5 of the 61 patients who took antibiotics actually harbored the gonococcus. Of these, all but one had an antibiotic-resistant infection, as compared with only 31% of the 121 patients who had not taken an antibiotic. More interesting, perhaps, was the finding that half the patients previously on an antibiotic had procured it through channels *other* than a health care provider. We cannot say whether the prior antibiotic use cured the majority of ingestors without detectable gonococcus or whether they never had infections. It is noteworthy, however, that so many were able to get the drugs without prescription— and in the United States at that. More importantly, the authors of this study concluded that, "the combined influences of relatively frequent self-administration of antibiotics . . . may have helped to accelerate the pace at which antibiotic-resistant *Neisseria gonorrhoeae* emerged in Baltimore."[2]

If antibiotics are "prescribed-only" drugs, how do individuals gain access to them? There are many ways, not the least of which is storing and using leftover drugs. When I ask people what they do with medicines they do not take, the vast majority respond that they keep them for later use. They do not find the question or the answer embarrassing, only curious. In any number of homes, should you open the mirrored bathroom cabinets, you'll find bottles of unused drug tablets and liquids. This is not uncommon. One family showed me some tetracycline that was outdated. There is not any guarantee of its effectiveness, let alone its safety. And in the case of tetracycline, as it ages, it converts to a chemical that could cause toxic liver damage if ingested.

A recent study in Spain revealed that almost half of a thousand randomly chosen households had bottles of unfinished antibiotics stored. However, in only 19% of the houses where antibiotics were found was there a person being treated. This finding is not unique to Spain. The antibiotics were probably deliberately saved or resulted from someone's failing to finish a prescription, a source of further misuse and selection of resistant strains.

People everywhere rely on antibiotics for different reasons—appropriately and inappropriately. Current practices do not always follow valid and prudent use, as the following examples will illustrate.

*   *   *

One woman came to the dermatology clinic at a local university-based hospital wanting treatment for a minor acne problem developing on her face. The resident physician informed her that the skin problem could be controlled by careful washing, proper skin care, and diet. There was no need for special medication. The patient became indignant and angrily demanded a prescription for tetracycline, a drug she knew by name because she had gotten it so many times before. The resident tried to explain to her why he advised against taking tetracycline for her minor skin problem. There was the risk of side effects, such as increased sensitivity to sunlight and a vaginal yeast infection. "But I want tetracycline," she exclaimed, pounding her fist on the clinic examining bed. The resident did not yield. Exasperated, the patient began screaming. "I want TETRACYCLINE . . . TETRACYCLINE!" which continued relentlessly despite attempts to calm her. Her shouts became even louder as the physician and nurse, embarrassed, hurriedly escorted her out (Figure 9.2, next page).

Clearly, this is an example of the extreme to which a patient might go in order to obtain an antibiotic. This patient's faith in tetracycline, coupled with her strong desire to clear up a flaw in her physical appearance, temporary as it was, led her to try to intimidate the physician into prescribing the medication. Under different circumstances, in another setting, such an action might have been successful.

*   *   *

A Washington businessman on his second plane trip to New York in three days felt a scratchiness in his throat. Without looking up from his work, he took a penicillin tablet out of the side pocket of his briefcase and swallowed it with his complimentary coffee. He was certain that this precaution would prevent his coming down with a full-fledged cold.

One pill would have no effect on an incipient throat infection, even if it were bacterial. In this case, it was probably a viral cold. Add to that his attitude, and that of the public in general, that such use is harmless. There is no concern for the side effects of such medications, worry about using drugs that are outdated, or fear of the selection of new resistant infectious agents. The problem is that, in most cases, no harm *is* evident and so the practice continues. Multiply this one instance by all those

Figure 9.2. Antibiotic misuse—the consumer demands. An insistent patient can be a problem to the physician and to the clinical establishment (Herbert Hächler, University of Zurich, Zurich, Switzerland).

individuals worldwide who keep antibiotics on hand and take them at the first symptom without physician advice and the magnitude of this indiscriminate use should become obvious.

*   *   *

A local real estate broker boasted that his mother has never had a problem getting any antibiotic she wants. "She first shops around until she finds a doctor who will write prescriptions for her."

A physician related a story relevant to this one. While he was looking after the patients of another physician who was on vacation, he was repeatedly asked by the patients to prescribe antibiotics for flu symptoms. When this covering physician refused because he did not think them necessary, the patients became upset. They complained to their own doctor when he returned. The covering physician was dismissed.

I recently asked a community physician about his experiences with antibiotic use on his own patients. "Patients ask for them by name," he replied. "It's tough not to give in to this pressure. Sometimes I do, sometimes I do not. It depends on how I feel about the situation and how I feel that day."

A doctor friend of mine in private practice outside of Boston related the following story. While being interviewed for a television show on antibiotic misuse, the TV crew began videotaping his interactions with different patients, all of whom agreed to appear on camera. One patient's visit is particularly compelling. A middle-aged woman with paper tissues in hand appeared in his office and sat down in an armchair in front of him. As the doctor began to take the history, which strongly suggested a cold, he asked to examine her, but said that he thought she had a viral cold. Without listening any further, the patient took charge. She interrupted, "Doctor, I know what I have and I know what I need. I want some ampicillin. And don't give me the 250mg tablets; they won't work. I want the 500mg pills."

This event may appear an exaggeration on the "patient demand theme," but it is a true story. It illustrates how much control patients want and how the antibiotic myth persists. If antibiotics were not by prescription, this patient would have obtained what she wanted. I have heard similar accounts from my colleagues. Of course, my doctor friend was placed in a difficult situation, but I'm pleased to say he did not give in. However, the patient never returned to see him.

As these examples illustrate, physicians complain that they have difficulty dealing with the demands of patients who persist in their beliefs that they need antibiotics. As noted earlier, sometimes the physician rationalizes that maybe there is a bacterial infection as well as the cold virus. And, if he gives in, he will prescribe a relatively "safe" antibiotic, like penicillin or tetracycline. While the drug, in general, may be relatively harmless to that patient, it will cause major changes in the bacterial flora associated with the patient and, indirectly, that of the environment. There is also the potential of side effects, such as diarrhea, rashes, and headaches, that certain individuals get with antibiotics. More general side effects, like nausea or stomach cramps, may also occur.

*   *   *

At a recent meeting of pharmacists, one local pharmacist relayed to me yet another chapter in the story of patient demand for antibiotics. He related that when physicians comply with patients urging them to provide the antibiotic, they often write the prescription for less than the therapeutic amount, thinking this action will be less harmful. I hope you now realize that such subtherapeutic usage will select against susceptible flora and propagate resistant strains, without treating the illness, most probably one that is not even present. In fact, the story represents two forms of antibiotic misuse—the drug was not needed and the dosage was not therapeutic.

Whom do we blame, the physician or the patient, when an antibiotic is obtained for a common cold? People welcome the report from the automobile mechanic that all their car needed was an adjustment or a new spark plug, but not a total motor overhaul. We do not argue about paying for his time and expertise. Why then should patients be disappointed when the doctor says that their viral diseases need only aspirin, fluids, and rest? There is a certain irony in this practice, since in "playing doctor," these people make decisions that potentially endanger their health and possibly their lives.

*   *   *

A mother of ten children told me how she keeps her family healthy. "I keep a stock of penicillin suspensions and tablets in case of earaches and sore throats." "Do you ever consult your physician?" I asked. "Only if the child doesn't get better in a couple days," she replied.

It was a revelation to her to hear that penicillin and other miracle drugs were not always miraculous. There was a great chance of missing the correct cause of the infection. It might not even be bacterial. If it were, use of the antibiotic could preclude identifying the true cause of the ailment. One could not determine whether the treatment was, at best, correct, or, at worst, a complication to curing it. The selection of resistant forms of bacteria in the household was not, of course, considered. She did not know that self-medication can be harmful and is often useless, certainly if an inadequate dosage is taken. And worse, it could help propagate a small amount of true disease agents into numbers large enough to cause infection.

*   *   *

A young mother in a Caribbean country witnessed her eight-year-old son being scratched by their cat. Although he was not upset, she became concerned about possible infection. She quickly loaded him into the car and headed to the doctor's office. There were fifteen people waiting ahead of her. "I wasn't going to wait." She told me. "He needed an antibiotic." So she went to a nearby pharmacy and obtained one. "Which one?" I asked. "I don't remember—one that the pharmacy had."

While we can understand the concern of the parent, we also see that she was taking her son's health into her own hands. What if the child had a reaction to the antibiotic? Perhaps she had chosen an antibiotic not to be used for children. Was an antibiotic really necessary? What about the possibility of a good scrubbing with soap, and a booster shot for tetanus?

*   *   *

On a plane trip to give a lecture in Illinois, I had an engaging conversation with my neighbor, who told me his child battled recurrent ear infections. He related that his four-year-old had been on low-dose amoxicillin every day for the past five months. I asked him when he planned to stop the medication. He replied that his doctor advised him to keep watch on the temperature outside (not of his child). When it was 63 degrees on 3 consecutive days, he could stop the medication.

As incredulous as this story may seem to some of you, others may recognize this as a personal experience. There are data from 20–30 years ago that show that chronic use of antibiotics, namely, ampicillin or amoxicillin, reduced the frequency of ear infections in certain children. But, in the face of resistance, recent data are not available. Clearly, the chronic use of an antibiotic at less than therapeutic amounts should select resistant mutants. If the approach works today, it is presumably not on the basis of antibacterial activity, but no studies are being done to examine this question.

*   *   *

In a visit to Harvard Business School to lecture on antibiotic use and abuse, I discussed the problem inherent in using tetracycline or erythromycin chronically for acne, a point we discussed earlier. Chronic, long-term use of antibiotics leads to selection of multiply resistant bacteria. I also discussed the other side of the problem. Namely, inadequate treatment, especially in terms of treatment of tuberculosis, can lead to selection of resistant strains. Following the lecture, a young female student came up to me to ask a question. She explained that she has been on daily tetracycline since age 16 for acne. She was now 22. I thought she was going to ask me whether she should now stop. Instead, to my surprise, she asked, "Do you think that I caused myself a problem when I forgot to take my medication for a few days?"

There are two points to discuss here. Firstly, is chronic use of an antibiotic for benign acne necessary? I am not speaking of a week or so, but extended to months and years. Secondly, even the brightest can miss the message. Surely inadequate treatment can be a problem for some diseases, but in the case of acne that is clearly not so. The long-term consequences to her immediate environment are the propagation and maintenance of resistant strains.

*   *   *

About 25 years ago, in Shiraz, Iran, a medical student was sent into 40 doctors' offices feigning a cold. He recorded not only the time in the office and the questions but also the final diagnosis. Thirty-four doctors diagnosed a viral illness, two an upper respiratory tract infection, and one a cold. The other three doctors found evidence for chronic or severe disease. While you may think that the latter misdiagnoses happen only in "that part of the world," reports from other countries have shown that this is clearly not true. But what was most important from the study was the treatment. Thirty-seven of the 40 physicians prescribed antibiotics, along with 12 other different types of medications including tranquilizers, calcium supplements, and sedatives. The bottom line is that the physician is often the culprit in the release of antibiotics for illnesses that are not of bacterial nature. This is an important area where improvement must be made.

Some 10 years later, I proposed doing a similar study of physicians in Boston and in Providence, RI. Unfortunately, my proposal was unequivocally turned down by the Human Investigational Review Board of my university. I was told it was unethical to put doctors under this kind of scrutiny. Someone even labeled it a "sting" operation. Following the publication of this book, I mentioned to others this study and my disappointment at not being able to do a similar study myself. While I was refused, FOX television's *FrontPage*, which did an extensive story on the problem of antibiotic resistance, performed the study on their own. The studio sent a 26-year-old assistant producer into four doctors' offices in Denver, CO, claiming that she did not feel well and relating symptoms of a cold. All four doctors prescribed antibiotics, and in each instance it was a different drug, two of which were third-generation medications.

The event prompts several questions. Why were the drugs prescribed? What were the signs that necessitated the prescription? Clearly they were only symptoms and not signs of illness since the patient was actually in good health. Why, in the same city, did she receive four different prescriptions? Only one physician agreed to be interviewed by the TV crew. He attributed his decision to treat on her history despite absent signs. He replied, "medicine is an art, not just a science."

Two other media groups performed the same type of study. The Canadian Broadcasting System sent a "patient" into 3 doctors' offices in Toronto with claimed "cold" symptoms— each physician prescribed an antibiotic. In a similar way, a member of Dan Rather's *48 Hours* team received antibiotics from two out of four Park Avenue physicians.

Although anecdotal, the reports are meaningful. In different places in North America, a prescription for antibiotics is relatively easy to obtain. The casual regard for antibiotics was illustrated as well in a 1998 *New Yorker* magazine cartoon. As a patient is leaving the office the receptionist says, "Don't forget to take a handful of complimentary antibiotics on your way out."

Changing Patterns of Antibiotic Use

The use of semi-synthetic penicillins, namely, ampicillin and amoxycillin, has risen over the last two decades in the United States.[3] This increase has occurred predominantly in the pediatric age group. The explanation for the increase is linked to the greater numbers of children attending day care centers, now that both parents typically work outside the home. In contrast to the times when children stayed at home or in smaller groups, the close child-to-child contact in these centers propagates the spread of common childhood diseases at earlier ages. This situation, antibiotic experts claim, has led to increased antibiotic usage. No one can be certain whether these illnesses are viral or bacterial, but antibiotics will be used often in any case. Thus, overall total annual antibiotic consumption goes up because it starts earlier and persists throughout the early years of school. This societal change puts additional pressure on the problem of selection of resistant bacteria. We do not criticize this change, but want only to increase awareness of its potential effect on the frequency of resistant infectious disease agents.

One research group in Texas compared the frequency of antibiotic resistance among children in day care centers with that of children staying at home.[4] The investigators made a remarkable, but perhaps not totally unexpected, finding. The level of resistant bacteria in the intestinal flora of the children in day care centers was at least twofold higher than that of children spending their days at home. Of particular interest, this higher level of resistance extended to relatively new antibiotics.

Antibiotics and the
Individual's Bacterial Flora

The infectious virulence of a bacterium is not changed by its being resistant. The only thing that changes is the bacterium's ability to take hold in the body if an antibiotic to which it is resistant has been used. Non-disease-causing bacteria are essential parts of the body's natural "armor" against invading infectious bacteria (Figure 9.3, next page). Once these are killed or diminished, resistant disease-causing bacteria can find a

Figure 9.3. *The bacteria lining the skin and intestinal tract form a protective "armor" against invasion by pathogens and other foreign bacteria. If, during antibiotic therapy, this protective coat is killed, resistant "invaders" have room to colonize and potentially cause disease problems (Bonnie Marshall, Tufts University School of Medicine).*

niche and multiply. Once they reach critical numbers, they can cause illness and, if resistant, will be harder to treat.

Our "protective" flora changes during the course of our activities and movements into new environments. We are constantly picking up and shedding bacteria. But these changes are of little or no consequence to our lives. If, during antibiotic therapy, we were to place ourselves within a germfree environment, bacterial exchanges with the outside would cease—we would be dealing only with our own bacterial flora. We could kill off all the susceptible microorganisms that we had and cause an increase only in the small numbers of resistant bacteria that were already there at the time the antibiotic was started. Once these resistant bacteria multiplied, reversion to a flora of susceptible bacteria would not be possible, since none could enter the germ-free environment. We could treat the resistant bacteria, if needed, with an appropriate antibiotic to which they were susceptible; however, we could do so without concern that other, resistant pathogenic bacteria would enter from the outside.

Obviously, the above scenario is, by and large, impractical; however, it is the reasoning now being applied in the treatment of cancer patients. When their bodies have become unable to cope with bacteria, they are placed in environments where entry of new bacteria is limited. These people are given diets of "cooked foods only," since these foods will be essentially free of bacteria. Living plants and flowers are removed from the rooms because bacteria that can potentially infect the patients may be present in them. By these means, we curtail the entry of infectious agents and we monitor the kinds of bacteria already there. Thus, we know what kinds of bacteria will potentially cause an infection or a new fever and have the appropriate antibiotics on hand to treat them, if needed.

For an otherwise healthy individual, taking prescribed antibiotics in the home and community is not hazardous. Rigorous precautions against bacterial pick-up, as used in very sick people, are not needed. The natural defenses are intact and the chance of meeting up with a dangerously large number of resistant disease-causing bacteria is small. Moreover, once the antibiotic course is finished, susceptible strains will eventually return.

The problem we face today is that even in the community, the numbers of susceptible bacteria are decreasing following the overuse of antibiotics. Thus, after an antibiotic treatment, the time for the return of the susceptible flora is greatly lengthened.

*   *   *

Lack of understanding of the difference between bacteria and viruses can affect antibiotic use. The public expects that antibiotics can treat viral colds. Confusion in the news media can be very influential to that effect. A 1996 article in the *Toronto Sun* described MRSA as both a bacterium and a "virus." The article went on to describe VRE as "a sometimes deadly virus." Said one senior nurse, "I think you can all surmise from the newspaper article that reporters and editors have a total misunderstanding of the difference between a bacterium and a virus. We have our work cut out for us."

*   *   *

At a medical meeting in Illinois a number of years ago, I asked physicians a few questions for anonymous electronic responses. Ninety percent said they had encountered patients demanding antibiotics. Perhaps most surprising was that 86% admitted having prescribed antibiotics against their better judgment.

The demand for antibiotics comes also to the pharmacy. In a 1994 report in the *Economist*, a pharmacist relates the events that occurred when antibiotics and other medications finally reached Vietnam. The customers wanted and demanded more than one capsule or pill for any illness. As we have discussed with doctors, the pharmacist, besieged with demands, wrestled with a quandary. "If I do not comply, the patient just goes to another pharmacist and I lose business."

The level of susceptibility of the returning flora after antibiotic ingestion will, as we have mentioned, depend on the source of that flora, be it the immediate environment or foods that we eat. One study in France showed that when people who had relatively high numbers of resistant bacteria in their intestinal flora ate diets of only sterilized foods, their intestinal flora became more sensitive.[5] These findings suggest that the resistant flora we have may come from the food we eat, or that selective substances (antibiotics?) are in the food that help propagate resistant bacteria.

Potential Individual Consequences of Antibiotic Use

Probably the most significant unwanted consequence to the individual taking an antibiotic is the side effects that are inherent in all drugs. The chance of a side effect can be as high as 50%, depending on the drug. Many of these side effects, however, are so mild that we accept them in exchange for benefits we receive from the antibiotic. When taking an antibiotic, most people can deal with a little abdominal discomfort—nausea, cramps—especially when it subsides after several doses of the drug. The skin rash from penicillins may cause us to stop taking the drug but is not inherently serious. Other side effects, however, can be quite severe and unexpected, such as the life-threatening allergic reaction to penicillin, which is rare but carries a 30% death rate with it.

Prolonged use of some drugs can lead to toxicity in critical internal organs. Gentamicin, an excellent antibiotic for treating systemic bacterial infections, can cause damage to the kidneys. Streptomycin, used previously for many infections of the intestine, kidney, and lung, and now used primarily, if not exclusively, for tuberculosis, can lead to hearing defects. In a report from China, one physician attributed a large percentage of hearing defects in children to the overuse of streptomycin and other drugs from the same antibiotic class.[6]

Another side effect of antibiotic usage is the overgrowth of one's natural bacterial flora by other bacteria, including ones that produce toxins. Diarrhea caused by overgrowth of *Clostridium difficile* in the intestine follows treatment with broad-spectrum antibiotics to which this microorganism is resistant. The patient, already sick with one disease, now begins to suffer from painful and sometimes life-threatening diarrhea. Fortunately, we still have another antibiotic available to treat this problem, which is, ironically, the consequence of other antibiotic use.

Often, after prolonged use of broad-spectrum antibiotics, such as tetracycline, a secondary infection with yeast may appear. This is what produces the itching and pain in the vaginal area experienced by women being treated with tetracyclines or penicillins for a variety of ailments.

An unexpected consequence stemming from antibiotic use was exemplified in the *Salmonella* outbreaks in the United States that we discussed earlier (Chapter 6). Those people who happened to be on antibiotics when they consumed either contaminated meat or milk came down with severe diarrhea caused by an antibiotic-resistant *Salmonella*. Under the selective environment of the antibiotic, the resistant *Salmonella* reached sufficient numbers to cause gastroenteritis and, in some cases, blood infections resulting in death. Most people not taking an antibiotic, who had ingested the very same contaminated products, remained healthy and unaffected.

There are precautions that a healthy person can take to prevent this indirect consequence of antibiotic ingestion, that is, the "pick up" and propagation of these resistant bacteria. For instance, one can wash meats and cook them well before eating them. Uncooked fruits and vegetables can be prepared on different kitchen surfaces than those on which raw meats and fish have been processed. Because cooking will kill the bacteria, it is the uncooked foods that serve as a bacterial cocktail. Even minor contamination of these uncooked foods with small numbers of resistant bacteria from meat or fish could allow enough viable microorganisms to be ingested and enter the body. Concurrent use of an antibiotic would help them to propagate and potentially cause disease.

Individual Efforts against
Antibiotic Resistance

We are at a point in medical history where people expect a "pill for every ill." Some of the reasons for this attitude we have already discussed. Antibiotics do not help unless bacteria are involved in the problem. It is anti*bodies* made by our bodies, not anti*biotics* made by molds and soil bacteria, that protect and control viral infections and also serve in protecting us against repeated bacterial invasion.

Faced with this situation and the knowledge of how resistant bacteria are propagated and spread, each individual can help curtail this mounting world health problem. First of all and most directly, the individual must understand what an antibiotic can and cannot do. Antibiotics are treatment moieties for bacterial infections, that is, infections caused by microscopic single-cell microorganisms that cause disease when they get inside the body. These microorganisms disrupt normal physiological processes and can eventually lead to death. Antibiotics are superbly unique in being able to kill the bacteria while producing relatively little harm to the body of the ingestor, whether an animal, human, or plant.

An individual should know when, why, and for how long the prescribed antibiotic should be taken. He or she should ask these questions of the physician and then follow the directions for use. If the antibiotic is given to treat a bacterial infection, it needs to be taken for the entire course of therapy and not simply until the symptoms disappear. Resistant forms of the causative bacteria can emerge and increase in number if the drug is stopped before a treatment course is completed. Once these resistant forms are numerous, subsequent treatment with that antibiotic fails.

The existence of antibiotic resistance is hardly cause for total despair. Most antibiotics, even the older ones, can and do still have some effective uses today. They could have greater impact if the resistant strains were more outnumbered by the susceptible ones. The fear of resistance precludes the use of an antibiotic until the physician knows the infecting microorganisms are not resistant. This is a far cry from 20 years ago when just knowing what kind of microorganism caused the disease was enough to choose the appropriate antibiotic. Pharmaceutical companies, at least those that have remained in the anti-infective field, are still working hard toward discovering and developing new antibiotics. To a large extent, new antibiotics are being sought to circumvent resistance. Others are being derived to deal directly with the resistance mechanisms themselves. The ideal goal, from this point on, is for these new drugs to be used wisely and appropriately so as to limit the rate of selection and appearance of resistance.

Traditionally, antibiotic regimens last 5–10 days. New studies show how we can shorten the time that antibiotics must be taken in order to cure certain illnesses. As we have noted, many patients with uncomplicated urinary tract infections can be cured with only 1 to 3 days of oral antibiotic treatment. So, in this common community infection, short treatment works. Maybe there can be more examples like this, especially when given the appropriate antibiotic. This direction toward shorter courses would limit the environmental presence and selective effect these drugs would have on the emergence of multiresistant bacteria. New tests will allow physicians to diagnose infectious agents early enough to know exactly which antibiotic to use and for how long. Vaccine development can lead to prevention of diseases for which antibiotics are now needed.

Dramatic protection against *Hemophilus influenzae* type b infections, in particular meningitis, has been achieved by a new vaccine against the organism. A similar approach is being taken with a vaccine directed against a number of pneumococcal strains that cause invasive disease, including meningitis. The positive results from the vaccination program provide hope that vaccination will decrease the frequency of disease and consequently the need for antibiotics. Controlling the presence of these two major bacterial causes of ear infections will hopefully provide more confidence to physicians to accept the symptoms as viral and not bacterial. Antibiotics can be withheld at least initially.

In fact, even without the vaccine, recent studies show that withholding antibiotic treatment for 24–48 hours for ear infection did not harm the individual and, in fact, a large majority of the patients recovered on their own. Thus, the combination of vaccination against two of the major bacterial causes and the realization that at least half of the patients will recover even when there is a bacterial cause should lead to a decrease in the immediate need to prescribe antibiotics for ear infections. Obviously, one also needs to add the right consumer education to deter the demand for antibiotics.

There may be some untoward consequences from vaccination. I am not speaking of problems for the patient, but on microbial ecology. The microbial world "abhors a vacuum." Therefore, with the elimination of *Hemophilus influenzae* type b, the related, non-typable *Hemophilus* strains have taken their place in respiratory tracts of some patients. These bacteria are now principal causes of sinusitis. Furthermore, the organisms are multidrug-resistant and therefore difficult to treat. Still, sinusitis is far less dangerous than meningitis. So the benefit of vaccination far exceeds the risk.

The initial findings following the pneumococcal vaccine show a similar result. Following vaccinations, other invasive pneumococcal strains, not covered by the vaccine, have appeared. It is too early to know whether these strains will lead to severe pneumococcal diseases. If so, we shall return to the need for antibiotics, and presumably vaccines can be made against these as well. There is an important message here. Any time one makes an attack on the microbial world, there will be a countermaneuver resulting in ecological change—the elimination of one group of bacteria will lead to replacement by others. We should take care that they are not more undesirable than the ones we have.

Antibiotics remain effective agents in curing bacterial diseases. They have revolutionized medical therapy and are a major stalwart against infectious agents. But we must use them prudently and appropriately to curtail the rate of emergence of resistance to new drugs and prevent spread of resistance among totally unrelated bacteria. Once the antibiotics are in the hands of the patients, the patients assume the responsibility for themselves and their families. They must follow the directions for use. The consequences of antibiotic misuse come back to haunt the misuser as well as a multitude of innocent bystanders in the community, most notably other family members.

We have seen how individuals and communities have been ravaged by the consequences of irresponsible abuse of antibiotics. People worldwide are finally beginning to understand this problem and to deal with it. Producers, prescribers, and consumers are all taking a greater part in curtailing antibiotic abuse. By using these drugs effectively, each one of us protects the world population from the continued emergence and spread of resistance determinants. We must take responsibility for using antibiotics properly, since this will protect the future health of ourselves, our families, and our whole society.

chapter ten

The Antibacterial Craze

Among many events that characterized the close of the 20th century was the escalation in sales of antibacterial-containing household products. The public sought new ways to control what they saw as a threatening microbial world.

In common parlance, an *antibiotic* is a natural substance that inhibits the growth of other microorganisms. *Antibacterials* would be those substances whose action is limited to bacteria. Commonly now, "antibacterial" has taken on new meaning as a substance that is not ingested but added to household products, like soaps, dishwashing detergents, plastics, paper, and clothing. Antibacterials also appear in play toys for kids, cutting boards, mattresses, chopsticks, and even telephone pads (Figure 10.1, next page). An estimated 26 such products were available to the consumer in 1992. The *New York Times* reported that by the end of the decade over 700 products were marketed.

The major chemicals used as antibacterials are triclosan, triclocarban, and quaternary ammonium compounds. While not ingested, these are still compounds that inhibit growth of bacteria. Any substance of this sort can potentially select for bacterial strains that are no longer susceptible to it. While

Figure 10.1. *How clean should we be? A variety of household antiseptics and disinfectants, as well as toothbrushes, chopsticks, plastics, and cloths, now contain antibacterial chemicals that were formerly used chiefly in hospitals (Graham Jones and Bonnie Marshall, Tufts University School of Medicine).*

these and other antibacterials have been used to protect patients from spread of infections in hospitals, it is only in the last five years that they have been marketed in home products. This phenomenon is particularly upsetting since it comes at the same time that the home is progressively replacing the hospital for continued care of patients, who often return home from the hospital with intravenous drug treatment, including antibiotics. Many of these patients need protection from microbial diseases while still in a vulnerable state of health. If antibacterials are already used in the home, there is great likelihood that the bacteria there have become resistant to the very antibacterials we need to protect our patient. In other words, besides antibiotics, antibacterial-containing antiseptics (used on people's skin and other living tissue) or disinfectants (used on inanimate surfaces) can contribute to the selection and propagation of drug-resistant bacteria, (Figure 10.2, next page).

One of the basic tenants of infection control is hand washing, which started with the pivotal studies of Simmelweis in the mid-1800s. He showed that simply washing hands diminished sepsis of the mother following delivery of the baby. Hand washing has been shown to significantly lessen person-to-person spread of infections. While washing with soap and water is sufficient to remove the microbes, addition of an antibacterial agent, such as an alcohol, produces a significant additive effect by immediately killing the organisms being removed. What complicates the current hand and household disinfectant market is the addition of chemicals, such as triclosan and quaternary ammonium compounds, that, unlike alcohols, peroxides, and bleaches, do not act immediately but require prolonged contact (minutes not seconds) to work.

The average person washes his/her hands for 3–5 seconds, which is too brief to remove tightly bound microbes but does remove some viruses and bacteria, and sends them down the drain. In the hospital, the addition of a chemical like triclosan can be beneficial if used for the time period required for its activity—minutes, not seconds. But with suboptimal usage, the chemical additive serves no additional purpose. The effect of washing remains with the soap's ability to physically remove microbes. Used too briefly to be effective, antibacterial chemical products in homes remain as residues on counters and on hands at less than optimal concentrations. In this way, they can select for drug-resistant mutants. In comparing different antibacterial substances, we can distinguish them based on their speed of action and their propensity to remain as residues on the surface. An agent that works rapidly without leaving a residue will produce its effect in seconds, leaving the surface available for the return of natural microbes. Alcohol, chlorinated products, and peroxides fill this description. Most U.S. hospitals now use alcohol-based hand washes. Chemicals

Figure 10.2. *Antibiotics and antibacterials (antiseptics and disinfectants) can select bacteria resistant to themselves and to other drugs. Thus bacteria may become cross-resistant to antibiotics and surface antibacterials (Bonnie Marshall, Tufts University School of Medicine).*

that take longer to be effective and remain as residues can help those environments where protection for longer periods of time is needed, for example, on hands during repeated manipulations. The problem with residues, however, is that they are diluted down to less than effective doses which more easily select resistant microbes.

Also called "biocides," antibacterials were believed to act at multiple sites, especially at the high concentrations found in the cleaning product. With no specific target, the idea that bacteria could emerge resistant to them was considered untenable. However, studies in our laboratory demonstrated that one of the most popular chemical additives, triclosan, has a definitive target, an enzyme involved in the synthesis of the cell wall. A simple mutation in the enzyme renders the bacteria resistant to triclosan, even at relatively high concentrations. The recognition of a target and of resistant mutants heightened concern that the overuse of products containing this chemical will, in fact, lead to a changed microbiology in the home and to the propagation and overgrowth of resistant bacteria.

To make matters worse, multidrug efflux pumps that pump out antibiotics can also pump out these antibacterial chemicals. Such is the basis of resistance to triclosan by *Pseudomonas aeruginosa*, the organism that plagues immunocompromised patients, particularly those with cystic fibrosis—the organism pumps out triclosan so it is not able to inhibit cell growth. Mutants of *Pseudomonas aeruginosa* and *E. coli* can be easily obtained that show high resistance to triclosan and to different antibiotics, based on these multidrug efflux pumps. The findings warn that the use of these chemicals in the home could select for bacteria with *multidrug* resistance, including resistance to antibiotics. This is certainly not a desirable environment for a sick patient returning home for continued care (Figure 10.3, next page).

While in the past we have regarded the home as a haven, free of unfriendly resistant organisms, today this may not be the case. The increased use of these antibacterials in so many households applies great pressure on the normal bacteria living there, potentially evolving the microbiology of the home into one more akin to that of a hospital.

Besides triclosan, other biocides can select for antibiotic resistance. Research workers in Japan showed that laboratory mutants of a strain of methicillin-resistant *Staphylococcus aureus* (MRSA) with low-level resistance to the antibacterial benzalkonium chloride expressed a 10-fold higher resistance

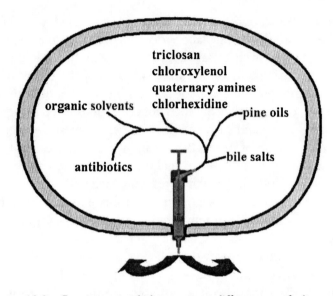

Figure 10.3. *Protein pumps which export many different types of substances (antibiotics, organic solvents, antiseptics, and disinfectants) protect bacteria from these toxic compounds (Andrew Prazar, Tufts University School of Medicine).*

to antibiotics, namely, penicillins and cephalosporins. The discerning feature of this laboratory experiment was that the mutants showed a drug resistance pattern strikingly similar to the new forms of MRSA that have recently been found in the community. As we discussed earlier, these MRSA, in contrast to those in the hospital, are still susceptible to most antibiotics, but resistant to penicillin and cephalosporins. To mark this distinction, microbiologists refer to them as community-acquired MRSA, or cMRSA. The findings raise questions as to the origin of the cMRSA. Did they emerge from the use of antibiotics in the community or from use of other agents—even perhaps an antibacterial? While purely speculative at the moment, the question invites studies to determine if there is such a link.

While producers of antibacterials claim that the products have been in existence for 30 years without causing a resistance problem, this was *limited* use, focused primarily in hospitals, not in homes. Now we are witnessing an enormous increase in application as homes throughout the U.S. and elsewhere in the world stock up on these products. Drug resistance emerges in response to increased amounts and durations of drug usage, a phenomenon poignantly illustrated by the history of antibiotics. Fluoroquinolone resistance was not a public health threat when this book was first published in 1992. It took time—years of misuse and overuse. The high-frequency resistance to the fluoroquinolones noted in *E. coli* at the end of the 1990s resulted from the increased usage of these drugs in communities throughout the world. Such an event was not expected at the outset since the drugs were so effective in killing the bacteria. Another example is the mounting resistance to vancomycin, not just in the enterococcus but in other genera, such as *Staphylococcus aureus* that have emerged with chromosonal mutations that produce vancomycin resistance. Again, this development has followed increased amounts and duration of vancomycin use.

In discussing the use of antibacterial products in the home, the important fact is the lack of demonstrated additional hygienic benefit from these antibacterials in the healthy household over normal conventional cleaning agents. The need and purpose for antibacterials should be the protection of the vulnerable patient—as has been provided in hospitals. When I send a cancer patient home for continued drug treatment, I suggest that the surfaces be wiped with products containing alcohols, bleach, or peroxides and that antibacterial-containing soaps be used in the care of these patients. However, I stress the need to use the latter for appropriate periods of time. The application is, therefore, for a designated medical need. If, however, these same products have been used in the house for regular cleaning then, stemming from our knowledge of antibiotics, I am concerned that the microbes in the home may have adapted to the antibacterials by becoming resistant. Then, the antibacterial product will not be effective in protecting sick family members returning home (Figure 10.4).

As we discussed earlier, overuse and misuse of antibiotics, let's say for viral illnesses, will render them useless as bacteria emerge with resistance. If we want to use antibacterials to protect patients from picking up infectious disease agents in the home, then we want active, effective agents. They will potentially not be effective if the same agents have been used in the home for general cleaning and not for a therapeutic purpose. We could have accepted a few such products on the market, but today consumers are hard-pressed to find home products that do not contain an antibacterial. Said one consumer "I cannot find anywhere, in any store, drug-free hand soap . . . this is insane." In fact, currently manufactured, some three-quarters of liquid soaps and one-third of bar soaps contain antibacterials. But the consumer only has access to what is displayed in supermarkets—largely if not exclusively the antibacterial-containing products.

The Hygiene Hypothesis

There is another concern stemming from the antibacterial craze. It relates to the recent rise in the frequency of allergies and asthmas. When the Berlin Wall and the Iron Curtain dissolved, allergists and immunologists looked at the newly "opened" countries, where air pollution was known to be high. They were surprised to find that the rates of allergies and asthmas were in fact lower than those among populations living in industrialized countries. This finding needed an explanation. It led to a reevaluation of the causes of asthma and

IT'S A QUESTION OF RESIDUES

Residues

Triclosan
QACs
Triclocarbon

Non-residues

Bleach
Peroxides
Alcohols

Figure 10.4. Antibacterials (or biocides) prevent transmission of disease agents to and from people. Bleaches, peroxides, and alcohols disinfect quickly and leave no residues. Others persist on surfaces where they become diluted and can potentially select bacteria resistant to themselves as well as antibiotics.

a changed paradigm. Clearly, air pollution was not the major factor. Unexpectedly, a consistent correlation appeared between excessive hygiene in the homes of people living in industrialized nations and increased allergy. The "hygiene hypothesis," touted initially by investigators in England and now receiving attention worldwide, associates overly hygienic living to faulty maturation of the human immune system.

A recent paper in the *New England Journal of Medicine* showed that children in daycare facilities with repeated childhood illnesses seemed protected against allergies later in life. One conclusion from this finding could be that we need to suffer through these illnesses or even try to acquire them to avoid health problems later. But the results do not necessarily mean that the organisms causing the illnesses are the reason for the protection. The illnesses may be merely markers of spread of harmless as well as harmful bacteria and viruses. The more abundant, friendly microbes are what are needed for the normal maturation of the immune system. In other words, like strengthening muscles and bones through exercise, contact with external microbes helps exercise our immune system to build our defenses against disease-causing microorganisms. If the immune system fails to "see" certain bacteria early, then the maturation of this defense system is faulty. Those at greatest risk are, of course, the infants and young children. If a balanced immune system is not formed, then the child responds later to various external environmental stimuli with asthma and other allergic responses. Interestingly, people immunized with the vaccine against tuberculosis seem to have a protection against allergy, apparently through the same mechanism—proper maturation of the immune system. An underlying fundamental event seems to be an infant's contact with various kinds of naturally occurring bacteria early in childhood, particularly bacteria living in soils and dirt, to protect against allergy later.

The new findings, which reversed the theory that allergy was due to air pollution, have led to a reevaluation of host response to the normal microbes we confront daily. The original studies compared homes that were overzealous in hygiene and food protection with those located in rural areas where such hygenic measures were much less. The findings reported reflect events that occurred *before* the current antibacterial craze. The now-added effect of antibacterials in homes only increases our concern about infants raised in those households. If the craze continues, we might expect to see an increase in the numbers of people with allergies—an adverse consequence seen much too late to make amends. Therefore, we should assess the situation now and evaluate any benefit with the potential risk.

The bottom line, of course, is whether antibacterials are really needed in the healthy household. As we have discussed before, there are no data showing they have any advantage over normal cleaning agents. The American Medical Association asked the FDA to evaluate and even regulate the use of antibacterial products in home products. This action was predicated on the finding that the substances can select resistant mutants and resistance mechanisms, some of which provide cross-resistance to antibiotics. To the latter concern we can now add the question of whether overuse of these products can change the kinds of helpful microbes in the home, leading to more allergies in the future. If these products are needed, as with sick patients, we can accept their use. The observed benefit exceeds potential risk and they are used for a definitive period of time—when patients are vulnerable. But, without such a need, and for what may be months to years of use, the risk is clearly unacceptable.

The antibacterial issue has captured the attention of the media worldwide. There is mounting interest in determining the true benefit of these products against the potential harm they may be causing. Investigators are beginning to find bacteria including MRSA, albeit at low numbers, with resistance to the antibacterials. So far, these isolates have come from hospitals. With unrestrained use of antibacterials in our homes, we may find a broader source of these resistant strains than we want or we anticipated.

chapter eleven

Antibiotic Resistance

*A Societal Issue at Local, National, and
International Levels*

Antibiotic resistance is not constrained by local or even national borders. It confronts all individuals and populations around the world. The answer to the problem must come from all societal groups. Misuse and overuse of antibiotics—whether in homes, hospitals, communities, animal populations, or agriculture—can provide the additional environmental force to select for and maintain resistant strains of bacteria (Figure 11.1, next page). The killing effect of antibiotics is so strong that only the resistant bacteria will survive. When it is the consequence of treatment, we can accept it, and it is usually transitory. But other uses of antibiotics exacerbate the resistance problem because they are inappropriate—namely, improper choice of an antibiotic and length of application.

To make matters worse, the resistance genes, harbored in one group of bacteria, can spread to vastly different types of bacteria and to areas far away. Resistant bacteria and their resistance genes do not need passports in order to cross country

275

Figure 11.1. Antibiotics are used as therapeutic drugs in many different areas. The principal ones are for people and for food animals, but another is agriculture. This usage includes home and hospital medications, growth promotion, prophylaxis, and therapy use in animals, and aerial treatments of plants and trees (Bonnie Marshall, Tufts University School of Medicine).

borders. They can quickly circumnavigate the globe, carried along as stowaways in humans, animals, and food products. This spread has been more rapid and insidious than anyone ever thought possible. Significantly, the resistant strains would have no survival advantage if there were no antibiotics present. Therefore, where use is limited, so are bacteria with resistance.

It is perhaps ironic and paradoxical that antibiotics, still the best agents for treating bacterial infections, are the single most important agents that select for and cause the propagation of bacteria resistant to them. This two-sided conflicting effect of these valuable drugs makes it crucial that we use them carefully.

Infectious disease experts have estimated that at least half of the human use of antibiotics in the United States, whether in the community at large or in hospitals, is unnecessary or inappropriate. Similar or higher levels of misuse have been documented in other parts of the world, but the actual extent of antibiotic misuse worldwide remains unknown. When this misuse is a superfluous use, there is an "extra" nontherapeutic selective force for the propagation of antibiotic-resistant strains.

Today, antibiotic resistance thwarts our ability to cure infectious diseases. The rise in multiresistance among bacteria, that is, the ability of a single disease-causing bacterium to resist more than one antibiotic, is steadily climbing to precarious proportions. Clinical strains of five different kinds of bacteria are resistant to all, or all but one of the available antibiotics. These include multidrug-resistant isolates of *Mycobacterium tuberculosis* (the cause of tuberculosis), *Acinetobacter baumanii*, *Pseudomonas aeruginosa*, vancomycin-resistant *Staphylococcus aureus*, and vancomycin-resistant enterococci. An approach to curb this tide is sorely needed. Let us recapitulate how antibiotics are presently being used and how we can best allay their ability to encourage the emergence and spread of resistant strains.

Availability to the Consumer

As noted before, in the United States and other industrialized nations, antibiotics for human treatment are to be obtained only through prescription. This regulation is applied to protect individuals from misuse and potential harm to themselves. Despite the need for obtaining a doctor's prescriptions, there are ways to get prescription medication if one wants it, such as by coercing one's physician or hoarding leftover medicines. Rather than bother with throat cultures, which can be done in the office and speedily examined for "strep throat," some doctors simply hand out prescriptions. In many instances, especially when the patient has no fever, the problem may be viral, not bacterial, and the antibiotics are useless. Such physicians are not helping their patients, and they are certainly not helping society cope with a burgeoning worldwide resistance problem.

As we have seen, for the majority of the world's population, antibiotics are available over-the-counter in pharmacies or from street vendors, as easy to obtain as aspirin and cough medicines. The patient does not need to visit a physician, wait for a diagnosis, or get a prescription. If the antibiotic is carried in the local pharmacy, the consumer can obtain it; however, only the few who can afford the costs of these drugs can take advantage of their ready accessibility. For this latter reason, while it is theoretically possible for the majority of the population to have easy access to these drugs, most cannot buy them. In the Dominican Republic, for example, one day's treatment with a penicillin derivative can cost more than the daily wage of a typical farmworker.

Whatever the means of distribution, the common denominator of antibiotic usage in all countries is the individual consumer. Therefore, any attempt to improve the use of antibiotics must focus on the person who asks for, buys, and takes the antibiotic. We can make great strides toward curtailing side effects and curbing antibiotic resistance if we can convince individuals that these drugs are not "cure-alls." Each person should take an antibiotic only when needed, that is, only when suffering from a known bacterial infection. These drugs are not meant to treat symptoms—they are not to be taken at the first sign of a sore throat or cough. People should understand clearly why they should not be stockpiling antibiotics in their homes to be given out to other members of the family or to neighbors.

Although antibiotics have been known and used for almost sixty years, people's attitudes toward them have changed very little. In the late 1950s, only twelve years after the success of penicillin and seven years after the discovery of the virtues of tetracycline and chloramphenicol, Henry Welch, then Director of the Division of Antibiotics of the U.S. Department of Health, Education and Welfare, stated in the New York Academy of Medicine's book *The Impact of Antibiotics on Medicine and Society:*

> The American public is like a huge sponge that absorbs antimicrobial agents like water, always eager to try the new one they have read about in their daily press or latest magazine, one whose miraculous cures emanated from the radio or television. It has reached the point where the physician can tell his patient—but he can not tell him much! The patient advises the doctor that he does not want antibiotic "A" because he has heard it is dangerous; he wants antibiotic "B" because a friend of his was cured with it. It makes no difference to him that his friend had an entirely unrelated infection. It's a "miracle drug"—let it perform its miracle.[1]

Has this opinion changed over these past forty-plus years? Such an attitude has persisted into the present decade, and without some broad effort to change it, it will continue into the next decade and beyond. We are paying the price for such misconceptions now in the form of unnecessary side effects and rapidly increasing medical costs.

We need to reeducate ourselves—we, the antibiotic-consuming public. We must alter attitudes that have their origins in the initial discoveries of antibiotics and their timeworn label as "miracle drugs."

Societal Consequences of Individual Misuse

Antibiotics are societal drugs. They are the only therapeutics that can bear this designation. Aside from the individual risks of side effects and allergies, there is a much larger societal effect stemming from widespread antibiotic use. This detrimental effect, however, is more subtle and certainly not one that is considered by the average individual who is taking the antibiotic. I am, of course, referring to the broad ecological changes that antibiotics produce. Antibiotic selection of resistant bacteria is environmental, not just individual. The appearance and propagation of resistant forms of bacteria pose a serious threat to society at large. Selection of antibiotic-resistant bacteria occurs in every user, wherever bacteria usually appear, such as in the intestinal tract, the mouth, and on the skin. We accept this consequence if the antibiotic is medically needed, but if not, the change in our bacterial flora is unnecessary and potentially harmful. These resistant bacteria can move to family members and to other people. While most of the resistant bacteria selected during antibiotic use are not those that cause harm to us, their resistance traits are often transferable. These bacteria have the potential to pass their resistance genes to harmful bacteria with which they come into contact.

A societal effect from antibiotics is set in motion every time we inappropriately use these valuable drugs. Not long ago I stated in an editorial, "Antibiotics are unique among pharmaceuticals in that they treat populations as well as individuals. One's bacteria are not solely one's own. Rather, they are shed, excreted, and otherwise spread into the environment, where they become part of a common pool."[2] In fact, the individual's flora probably reflect the environmental flora in which that person lives—the kinds of bacteria and the frequency of antibiotic resistance there (Figure 11.2).

Several years ago a dermatology group in England compared the skin flora of household dwellers of patients being treated with tetracycline, erythromycin, or cotrimoxizole for acne with a cohort of households that did not have treated acne patients. There was a highly significant increase in the numbers of resistant bacteria on the skin of the household contacts of the acne-treated patients as compared to the control group. Thousand-fold differences in multidrug resistance

Figure 11.2. *The bacteria associated with each individual may reflect common bacteria in the immediate environment and, in turn, society. Antibiotics can dramatically affect this societal microbiota (Herbert Hächler, University of Zurich, Zurich, Switzerland).*

were demonstrated.[3] This phenomenon is not one we would expect from any other therapeutic.

A study that examined the frequency of antibiotic resistance in intestinal *Escherichia coli* bacteria is also pertinent to this point. The investigators determined the numbers of resistant *E. coli* in the feces of infants and small children in three geographically distant cities on three different continents: Caracas, Venezuela; Qin Pu, China; and Boston, Massachusetts.[4] The investigation unveiled a number of important findings. First, in all three cities the majority of the children being considered for the study groups had already received an antibiotic, even though most were under five years old. Among the several hundred interviewed, fewer than 10% had not taken an antibiotic, and this included a majority of infants. Focusing on those children who had not received an antibiotic, the examiners assayed the numbers of *E. coli* in their intestinal tract showing resistance to eight separate drugs. In Boston, very few of this small subgroup of infants had *E. coli* that were resistant to any of the drugs; in those children who did, the resistant *E. coli* were present in low numbers. In the other two cities, however, the flora of the infants showed large numbers of resistant and multiresistant *E. coli*. Why the difference? The investigators have not yet fully answered the question, but one difference was clear from the outset of the study—antibiotics are obtained more easily and used more frequently in Venezuela and China than in Boston. These findings suggest that the total societal use of antibiotics may determine the native flora of each individual in that society.

We can look into this question another way. Infants are born sterile, that is, without any bacteria. They have come from a sterile environment, namely, the womb of the mother. Once introduced into the environment, their bodies are quickly colonized by bacteria with which they have contact. This change begins with the birthing room and the mother. The relative frequency of resistant and susceptible forms of bacteria that they acquire at birth will depend on what is most frequent in that environment. They are, in a sense, barometers of their immediate "bacterial environment," *until* they begin taking antibiotics themselves. Once on antibiotics, they become part of a process of bacterial selection that will push the flora to even higher levels of resistance.

The authors of this *Escherichia coli* study proposed a goal for the future—a low "resistance index." If, as they showed, we start out life with low levels of bacterial resistance, let's strive to maintain this "resistance-free" state. One clear goal is to reduce the reservoirs of resistance genes in the environment. And one means to do this is to improve the ways in which antibiotics are being used.

A recent study in Nepal further illustrates this point. A Tufts medical student, Judd Walson, determined the antibiotic resistance frequency of bacteria in the intestines of ambulatory people living at increasing distances from the capital city of Kathmandu. Through interviews and observation, he related the consumption of antibiotics by the individuals in these different communities with the levels of resistant bacteria in their intestines. He noted that the frequency of antibiotic resistance reflected more the availability of antibiotics in the total community than the consumption of antibiotics by the individuals in that community. A society with easy access to antibiotics, such as exists in Kathmandu, produces a higher frequency of antibiotic resistance among its people. Lower levels of resistance were found in people living in communities at a distance from Kathmandu, where health care facilities were far less accessible and the density of people was less, although the individual use of antibiotics was the same.

A similar conclusion came from studies of the frequency of resistant pneumococci in different communities in Spain. The studies reflect what I call the "selection density"—the amount of antibiotic provided to the number of individuals (people, animals, trees) in a specific geographic setting.[5] Obviously, the denser the population of treated individuals the more prominent will be resistant strains and their ease of spread and the harder it will be for a susceptible flora to survive and compete. The same phenomenon holds true in daycare centers where, during cold season, a large proportion of the children in close proximity are taking antibiotics and sharing their resistant flora.

As soon as we entered the antibiotic era, microbiologists and clinicians began to notice bacterial resistance. The problem was first evident when penicillin-resistant staphylococci appeared in hospitals in England and subsequently were tabulated throughout the rest of the world. The full implications of resistance, however, were not realized until the last three decades. Seemingly overnight, doctors discovered that they could no longer cure common illnesses with conventional antibiotics. This problem was as evident in the general community as in the hospital, where children's acute ear infections, skin infections, and pneumonias remained unaffected by penicillins. Resistance traits had appeared in community-acquired bacteria that had previously been uniformly susceptible to antibiotics. This change was the direct consequence of the tremendous selective power of antibiotics for resistant types of bacteria. Additionally, there was the unexpected presence in the environment of genes already available to the microbial world that rendered bacteria resistant and that could be exchanged among them. Exacerbating this situation is the widespread attitude of the public. "So what if I take an antibiotic? What harm can it do?"

In most instances, this indirect consequence, that is, selection of a resistance trait or a resistant bacterium, may not affect a particular person at the time, but it potentially compromises the future antibiotic therapy of family members and neighbors. More directly, however, the ingestor can be put at risk. Patients under treatment for cancer, as we have noted, become more susceptible to infections and can contract diseases even from the normal bacteria colonizing their own skin and intestinal tracts. If these strains are resistant, even if they do not normally cause disease they can become life-threatening because of the patient's weakened condition, and because the resistance of these microorganisms circumvents treatment.

As people continue to misuse antibiotics, more resistant bacteria with different kinds of resistances are surfacing, and, in turn, newer and more expensive antibiotics are needed to treat them. We may reach a point where costs preclude availability. What will we do then? It is time for all of us to deal with the rising problem of resistance and correct the public's misconception about the all-encompassing power of antibiotics. We need to convince ourselves, and those seeking out these drugs, that antibiotics have a defined role in medical

Figure 11.3. Let's make peace with the commensal bacteria and allow them to outcompete and replace resistant strains (H. Hächler, University of Zurich).

therapy. By taking them inappropriately, we expose ourselves, as well as the rest of society, to life-threatening risks.

As we enter the new millennium, we should change our approach toward bacteria. We should give up war and come to the peace table (Fig. 11.3). Our biggest allies are the commensal bacteria, those that help us and do not cause disease. They can outcompete the resistant strains that we have propagated by our overuse of antibiotics. As we begin to use antibiotics more prudently and in a more environmentally neutral way, we can revive the commensal flora of susceptible strains, which can then replace the resistant ones.

Who Provides the Antibiotics?

Putting the individual consumer aside for the moment, we should understand the role of the physicians, veterinarians, dentists, pharmacists, and government health officials who distribute these antibiotics. These prescribers represent a critical link in the chain leading from antibiotic production to antibiotic use and finally to antibiotic resistance. In developed countries, patients have little formal access to antibiotics without proper prescriptions. Thus, this group of prescribers holds the power to provide sound judgments in the dispersal of antibiotics. Yet, some will dispense antibiotics on demand by the patient or prescribe them as substitutes for other remedies that would have been just as effective and less risky. Antihistamines, fluids, and antiinflammatory agents are all that is needed for the relief of symptoms of the common cold.

In developing countries, however, such professional groups are not the primary dispensers of antibiotics. This role is often played by the local pharmacy. There are a number of reasons for this situation, not the least of which is the number of available physicians. While there is, on the average, one physician for every 520 people in industralized countries, this number is about one for 2,700 in most of the developing world, and the ratio can reach 17,000 patients per physician in the least-developed countries. With so few physicians available, other ways of obtaining necessary drugs, including antibiotics, needed to be established. Thus, antibiotics are available through the pharmacy without a prescription or they can be bought through the black market. To some extent, the ease of procuring antibiotics relieves some of the problems created by the paucity of medical personnel for these people. Still, a safe balance between the health needs of the people and the efficacy of antibiotics must somehow be realized.

While over-the-counter sales have been one solution to the problem of too few doctors, the situation has created menacing results. The easy availability of antibiotics has contributed to the emergence and spread of resistant strains so that readily accessible drugs no longer cure common infections. Yet these antibiotics continue to be used. Consequently, rather than kill off the disease-causing agents, they enable them to thrive in the patient and spread easily to others. Money is wasted on ineffective medicines that could have been used to buy food or clothing.

A group from Nigeria, evaluating the rising frequency of antibiotic resistance there, spoke out on the need for newer antibiotics to treat common disease agents in the face of a high frequency of multidrug resistance to the older antibiotics. They explained,

> Health policies in most developing countries include some form of National Formulary leading to the purchase of a restricted range of drugs. In the case of antibacterials, this most likely means that the greater proportion of available funds is spent on the purchase of older and cheaper agents. But is this wise, in view of the high prevalence of strains that are now resistant to these agents? It undoubtedly looks sensible on the budget sheets, but would the average householder consider it a "good buy" if a new brand of detergent powder, marketed at one-third the price of other brands, carried a 60% or more chance that the packet contained sand instead of detergent? Probably not. And the same would seem to be true when older, cheaper antibiotics are given to patients without the sensitivity of the infecting organism being known. The householder would want to look inside the packet before it is purchased for use. Older antibiotics may be a waste of money, despite being cheap, unless it is also possible to "look inside the packet," by having facilities for bacteriological testing, before they are used.[6]

The same view was voiced by examiners of antibiotic use in Costa Rica.[7] Here, resistance to ampicillin (a penicillin derivative) in many gram-negative pathogens was so high that the drug was hardly useful. The situation led to the removal of ampicillin from outpatient pharmacies and the addition of newer, albeit more expensive, drugs to deal with these resistant microorganisms.

Given the poor health care delivery in developing countries, solutions are not easily envisioned, but some can and should be considered. For instance, certain antibiotics could be made available to the people by governments expressly to treat the major diseases or epidemics affecting that population. Acute respiratory tract bacterial infection is a common disease affecting infants and children in less-developed countries. Treatment failure in this illness often means death. In making the choice of the right antibiotic, decision-makers need to know the major disease agents in their areas and the antibiotic susceptibility of these bacteria. With this information, they could focus their limited budgets on just those particular antibiotics that are active against the recognized disease-causing agents known to exist in that region.

The government of Cuba took just this kind of stand in the face of rising antibiotic resistance. It removed all of the recent generation drugs from the outpatient pharmacies and put them under the control of the hospitals. While antibiotics are not readily available in Cuba, the newer ones are now reserved for hospital physician decisions, not community physicians or over-the-counter availability. In this way, the misuse of some of the newer drugs, and subsequent resistance emergence, have been controlled and valuable antibiotics are reserved for the seriously ill hospital patient.

A limited number of drugs could thus be made available, namely, those known to be effective for the disease at hand in a particular locale. Others, even the more expensive antibiotics, could be reserved for drastic problems of resistance. Such an approach would remove the need for supplying many different kinds of antibiotics. It would hold newer antibiotics in reserve that could be used to treat only those patients harboring otherwise untreatable antibiotic-resistant infections. This approach would impart availability and effective use, despite limited public health monies in these countries. Such a rational system should bring more antibiotics, and, more significantly, the *right* ones, to areas where underuse and misuse of the drugs, *not* overuse, undermine medical therapy of the population.

Underuse Has Unfortunate Consequences

In the developing world, large numbers of people are at risk of dying from acute bacterial respiratory and systemic diseases, either because adequate therapy is not obtainable or because the drugs available are not effective. Large numbers of appropriate antibiotics are needed to treat these individuals, who are often impoverished and unable to pay for a visit to a physician, let alone the cost of a course of antibiotics.

For many patients served in primary health care clinics in developing countries, a single dose of an antibiotic is all that is available or affordable. Paradoxically, this minimal treatment allows the illness to flourish. A study of antibiotic usage in a refugee camp on the Thai border, reported by a paramedic from the United States, illustrates this situation.[8] Over one-third of the patients received only a single antibiotic dose despite serious bacterial illnesses. The same paramedic also reported how antibiotics were stolen from local pharmacies and clinics and sold on the "black market" to people who could afford them and who then used them as they saw fit.

I personally have seen antibiotics, made attractive by their colorful capsules, sold in small plastic sacks in markets in Nairobi, Kenya. The source of these capsules and their effectiveness were not readily known. This kind of easy availability fosters gross misuse, which in turn propagates resistance and unsuccessful treatment both for the person and the community. In Bangladesh, as of 1990, over 80% of *Shigella dysenteriae* type 1, the cause of bloody diarrhea, were resistant to ampicillin or trimethoprim/sulfamethoxazole or both, agents of first choice in the treatment of this disease. Multidrug resistance was characteristic of *Shigella* of all types found there, as is also the situation in Vietnam, Africa, and South America. The leading culprit is not the antibiotic itself but its use or misuse. As one infectious disease expert explained, "Insufficient quantity or multiple antimicrobial agents are given simultaneously. Often antimicrobial agents are given when there is no indication for use."[9] How does this occur? As we discussed elsewhere, it is through easy availability in private pharmacies without the need for a physician's prescription (Figure 11.4).

In Southeast Asia, Latin America, and other less-developed areas of the world, 70% to 80% of the patients who go to the local clinics have infectious disease problems that need antibiotic treatment. In a study conducted in Aceh Province in Indonesia in the mid-1980s, primary health care physicians reported that 65% of consecutive outpatients received or were prescribed antibiotics.[10] About a quarter of these patients purchased only half the amount of the antibiotic prescribed. This is presumably because of the high price they had to pay, along with the mistaken impression that just small amounts of these drugs were necessary to cure them of their diseases. In a similar analysis performed at about the same time, 70% of the patients attending an outpatient clinic in Santo Domingo, Dominican Republic, suffered from infectious diseases, predominantly caused by bacteria. Again, the economic constraints of the clinic gave the physicians there only enough antibiotic for the first day's treatment. The rest was to be filled by a prescription. About half of the patients never filled their prescription. They could not afford it. In all these examples, less than optimal antibiotic treatment is provided. This practice leads to failure to cure, as well as selection and propagation of resistant bacteria.

Figure 11.4. *Over-the-counter sales in developing countries make antibiotics easily accessible to those who can afford them. This private pharmacy in Bangladesh claims to have the answer for all illnesses. It is this type of availability of antibiotics that many believe contributes largely to the propagation of resistant bacteria (Michael Bennish, Department of Medicine, New England Medical Center, Boston, Massachusetts).*

Perhaps the clearest example where drug underuse has propagated resistance is in the treatment of tuberculosis. The tubercle bacillus hides in places in the body where the drugs do not penetrate well. Treatment usually requires six months of daily antibiotics. Incomplete treatment leads to inadequate eradication of the organism, leaving alive those bacteria that are inaccessible or the least drug susceptible. With the drugs gone, the surviving bacteria begin to multiply again and the disease returns with a vengeance in a form that is often resistant to the drugs previously used. What happens with the tuberculosis organism can happen with other bacteria that can hide in cells of the body, like the organisms which cause pneumonia.

Persistence of Resistance

While we know that antibiotic usage has contributed to the selection of resistance genes, we do not understand what causes the sustained, relatively high levels of these resistances in areas and countries where the antibiotic has been stopped. Since this persistence is not associated with the constant presence of an antibiotic, it presumably relates to other features of the resistance phenomenon. We also know that there is a slow loss from the environment of previously selected antibiotic resistance determinants.

To understand the phenomenon, we should take a look at the total picture. After a period of antibiotic selection, there exists a resident population of bacteria that harbors resistance genes. These bacteria are not very different from the other bacteria usually found in these environmental niches, except that they bear resistance traits. When the antibiotic is removed, these bacteria remain because they have now become a major component of the normal microbial flora. There is no factor or agent selecting *against* the resistant bacteria. These features probably contribute to the persistence of these genes in bacteria normally resident in that ecological niche.

But there may be other contributing factors. Many resistant bacteria also carry genes for resistance to heavy metals, such as mercury. Recent evidence suggests that mercury is a common environmental contaminant.[11] This fact may be especially true in the human body, where tooth fillings bearing mercury are almost universally present and from which small amounts of mercury are released on a daily basis. Enough mercury predictably flows through the intestine to select for mercury-resistant bacterial strains. If these strains also bear antibiotic resistance genes on the same plasmid or in the same bacteria as those with mercury resistance, then the mercury serves to maintain antibiotic as well as mercury resistance in that environment and in these bacteria. In other words, one growth-inhibiting agent, in this case mercury, can select for mercury-resistant bacteria that carry resistance to other growth-inhibiting agents, namely, antibiotics. All the resistances have found their way into the same bacteria and often onto the same plasmid. This is the same phenomenon we discussed before in regard to one antibiotic being able to select for plasmids with resistance to other antibiotics.

The Critical Role of Industry

The pharmaceutical manufacturers play a crucial role in the development and delivery of antibiotics. Most, if not all, of the major antibiotics currently in use have been developed through the auspices of the pharmaceutical industry. These companies had considerably fewer capital assets when they took on the development of penicillin in the early 1940s than they do now. That risky undertaking paid off and helped form the foundation of what is now a multi-billion-dollar industry. Their efforts have brought major antibiotics into production and have made them available for the treatment of serious illnesses around the world. Like some physicians and other antibiotic dispensers who sometimes prescribe antibiotics inappropriately, however, the pharmaceutical industry has contributed to antibiotic misuse problems as well.

Marketing techniques for antibiotics made in one country that are then sold in another are often inconsistent, and, in some cases, are simply unethical. For example, some citations for antibiotics claim broader uses for people in one country than for people in another country. More importantly, all of the possible side effects are not listed on the package inserts in the antibiotic preparation. Many more precautions are listed for antibiotics sold in the United States than in less-developed countries. Such inconsistencies have fostered unrest among consumer-based organizations that carefully examine products being introduced into their markets. When questioned, manufacturers often defend their actions by stating that they are only adhering to the regulations of the particular country. While this response may be true, consumer groups argue that this attitude is not ethical when dealing with human health. The problem here is that some countries are less demanding than others in these matters. The potential for and severity of side effects should be printed on every drug label, and provided as a standard in all countries, regardless of local regulations. The International Association of Pharmaceutical Companies advocates this principle, but discrepancies still exist. As a best case, it would seem fitting that the individual companies monitor their own practices.

Direct confrontation, legal actions, and the printed word from consumer organizations have brought these issues out into the open for the public to review. These consumer groups raise important questions and demand immediate answers. The groups include: Health Action International (HAI), which is an umbrella for many consumer organizations worldwide; the International Organization of Consumer Unions (IOCU); Social Audit in England; and Medical Lobby for Appropriate Marketing, Inc. The latter group has succeeded in getting several ineffective or potentially harmful drug combinations withdrawn. It has engineered the removal of drugs from certain combinations because they were superfluous and not useful. In other areas, misleading advertising claims have been modified. It is reassuring that, in many instances, industry representatives have responded to these concerns by either explaining their rationale, removing or altering the product, or changing the package insert description.

The Cost of Antibiotic Resistance to Society and the Individual

Certainly the most critical consequence of antibiotic resistance is the compromised therapy of human disease. Another mounting and disturbing consequence of resistance, however, involves the price tag for treatment. Someone must pay for the higher costs of newer drugs that are needed to combat resistant bacteria. Medical insurance companies, the government, and the individual now face, and will continue to face, higher and higher prices for the new antibiotics being developed to treat the multiresistant forms of bacterial disease. Some of these drugs can cost over $500 a day for treatment! Consider that price next to a cost of less than a dollar a day for some older forms of penicillin. One investigation from the United States Centers for Disease Control and Prevention reviewed 175 published and unpublished accounts of hospital- and community-acquired bacterial infections. They concluded that, for infections in the hospital and the community, "The mortality, the likelihood of hospitalization and the length of hospital stay were usually at least twice as great for patients infected with drug-resistant strains as for those infected with drug-susceptible strains of the same bacteria."[12] The inability to treat effectively a resistant infection immediately in an elderly patient may mean a greater chance of death than if the bacteria were susceptible; the same is true for a child. Timing is important in the struggle to prevent the bacteria from overwhelming the patient.

Another study used different mathematical models and assumptions to arrive at the actual costs of resistance to society. Depending on whether or not death was a consequence, the total societal costs of antibiotic resistance ranged from $150 million (without deaths) to $30 billion (with deaths) each year in the United States alone.[13] This study tried to factor in, as well, the effect of a resistant infectious agent appearing in one year on the cost to society in later years.

The 1995 U.S. Office of Technology Assessment report attributed $1.3 billion (1992 dollars) a year for infections caused by resistance in six species of bacteria in U.S. hospitals. Other data, comparing methicillin-resistant (MRSA) and susceptible

Staphylococcus aureus (MSSA) in New York hospitals estimated that treatment of each MRSA-infected patient costs 6–10% more than treating one with a susceptible strain—about $2,500 to $3,700 more per MRSA-infected patient. The total extra cost annually for treating the almost 3,000 MRSA-infected patients ranged from $7 to 10 million in just one city.[14] For tuberculosis, drug resistance means a hundred-fold higher cost for drugs than treatment of a susceptible organism. This could amount to $2,000 to treat each tuberculosis patient. These costs of resistance are estimated. We need more studies to demonstrate the economic impact of resistance. Such information will help convince local and national governments to support more work on antibiotic resistance. Further, what is not quantified is how resistance may increase the spread of inadequately treated infections in semi-closed environments like the hospital.

In developing countries of the world, the additional costs for new medication cannot possibly be met and, thus, these new, more costly antibiotics are not available there. Individuals living in the developed world are also fortunate in having excellent public health conditions that curb the incidence and spread of infectious diseases. Most of them have the ability to pay the higher price of newer drugs when faced with antibiotic resistance. This option is not open to the less fortunate people living in developing, and often more populous, areas of the world. We must also consider the cost to the pharmaceutical companies of developing new antibiotics to treat these resistant bacteria. Hundreds of millions of dollars are invested in the discovery, development, and animal and human testing of new antibiotics. This procedure takes years—a mean of ten years—as well as great sums of money. We have neither the time nor the money to spare. These mounting monetary and time constraints have provoked some companies to abandon the field of antibiotic research altogether—a decision that poses further detriments to society.

Once tested and approved, an antibiotic enters the market. Herein lies the conflict between research, development, and marketing. The company, its board members, and stockholders want to recuperate their investment—the sooner the better in this competitive field. To do so, the company must advertise the new antibiotic to physicians and sell it in pharmacies. How much of the cost should be returned in the first year? The second year? If there is concern about an upcoming competitive drug, the pressure to sell as much as possible, as soon as possible, will be heightened immediately. No one can blame the pharmaceutical sales agents for encouraging the use of their product—within reason. The control on its choice and usage, however, must be at the level of the provider (hospital pharmacy, government health officer, health plan officer) and consumer. If the medical need is met by the new drug and the advantages over older, less-expensive agents are clear, then the new drug should be purchased and used. Yet, where less-expensive, older agents can be used, would it not be wiser to use these? While the pharmaceutical house may receive less revenue in a single year, the time between drug introduction and the emergence of resistant bacteria will be lengthened. This will provide the pharmaceutical company with a longer "run" for the product. And the cost to the entire health care industry will be lessened.

Problems in the Developing World

While the numbers of people in the United States suffering from antibiotic-resistant infections are increasing, they are relatively small when compared with the much larger numbers of people in less-developed nations who become infected with common resistant pathogens, those causing diarrhea or pneumonia. None of us who has followed the resistance problem will forget the thousands of lives lost in Central America in the 1970s when a multiresistant *Shigella* could not be touched with the available antibiotics. Resistance was still a curiosity and the consequence was brought home clearly in this epidemic. Some physicians were convinced they were dealing with an amoebic parasite causing the diarrhea—they had never confronted such a resistant bacterium. The epidemic of dysentery in Zaire in the early 1980s was also caused by a multiresistant *Shigella dysenteriae*. Hundreds lost their lives from an infection that should have ordinarily responded to antibiotics and fluid therapy. Such a situation could conceivably emerge in the developed world if we continue on our present path. We noted earlier the approximately 100 deaths a few years ago in Tajikistan from typhoid fever caused by multidrug-resistant *Salmonella typhi*. Let us not forget the problem with multiresistant staphylococci in the hospitals of Melbourne, Australia.

The Animal Issue

The use of antibiotics as growth-promoting agents in livestock has generated heated controversy in the United States and Europe for several decades. Whereas Europe responded in the 1970s by banning any antibiotics being used for humans from being used in feed additives, the United States Food and Drug Administration has not. The Natural Resources Defense Council, whose mandate includes wide environmental issues, adopted the animal feed problem as one of its investigational issues during the 1980s. It filed legal briefs with the Food and Drug Administration, including its famous 1985 "Imminent Hazard" petition that it placed before Margaret Heckler, then secretary of Health and Human Services. This latter document pointed to a large number of deaths from *Salmonella* infections linked to animal products, and associated the effect of antibiotic usage at any level with the emergence of resistant *Salmonella*. Margaret Heckler rejected the petition on the basis of lack of evidence for an "imminent" hazard, but, quoting Frank Young, the FDA Commissioner, she allowed the possibility of the issue to be revisited when more data had been accumulated.

The issue did, in fact, eventually come before a committee formed by the National Academy of Sciences' Institute of Medicine a few years later. This highly esteemed group of experts examined only the risk of death from use of antibiotics in animal feed. Because of limited data on other microorganisms, they focused on *Salmonella* as the causative agent. Thus, they left out the general issue of morbidity and the specific consequences of other disease-causing agents such as *Listeria* or *Campylobacter* or even *Escherichia coli*. This group, reviewing past and new data, concluded that although the committee was "unable to find a substantial body of direct evidence that established the existence of a definite human health hazard in the use of subtherapeutic concentrations of penicillin and the tetracyclines in the animal feeds . . . [nevertheless] the committee believes that there is indirect evidence implicating subtherapeutic use of antimicrobials in producing resistance in infectious bacteria that cause a potential health hazard."[15] But they were unable to assign a clear value factor to the risk. This inexactitude stems from the inability to assess which kind of use, therapeutic or growth-promoting, led to the emergence and propagation of resistant bacteria.

As discussed earlier, the Center for Veterinary Medicine of the U.S. Food and Drug Administration has mounted a comprehensive effort to control how antibiotics are provided to animals in terms of potential impact on human health. The Framework Document, which separates antibiotics into categories based on their value to human medicine and rationale for animal use, is under discussion by the agency with the industry and the public. In early January, 2001, experts at a three-day session in Washington, DC, attempted to define certain thresholds of antibiotic resistance in bacteria coming from animals that would predict potential problems of antibiotic resistance in humans. Although no decisions were made, those groups present urged that the same principles for prudent use of antibiotics be practiced in animals as it is being promulgated in people. The recently released FAAIR project report from the *Alliance for the Prudent Use of Antibiotics* is another additional technical report for use in these ongoing discussions.

In 1992, when this book first appeared, little seemed to be happening to deal with the concern of resistance stemming from antibiotic usage in animals, in particular for growth promotion. It is reassuring to know that now there is activity by world and national government and non-government groups to resolve some of the questions surrounding the use.

We expect that the debate on the use of antibiotics for growth promotion will continue as more data are accrued. Perhaps, as we are now seeing, the issue will die out because farmers are voluntarily withdrawing antibiotics and replacing them with nonantibiotic alternatives or other more natural farming methods. The public has become a powerful lobby— asking for meat and agricultural products that are untainted by resistant bacteria, antibiotics, or other chemicals.

Resistance Viewed from the World Perspective

The problem of resistance is multifaceted in its origins and manifestations, but we can still surmount it. Although resistance is clearly an international problem and the demographics of language and mentality may be different in each country, there are similarities in the profiles of all members of society prescribing and consuming antibiotics everywhere. It is the relative numbers of each antibiotic user and prescriber type that may be different, depending on the country and its number of medical personnel. The universal features of this widespread problem have convinced individuals and groups in countries worldwide to take an active role in solving it. Countries on all continents are becoming increasingly aware that antibiotic resistance is not a problem unique to their country or even their continent. There need be no embarrassment that resistance has emerged in their country—bacterial resistance is a global dilemma.

A group of over 100 experts from more than 30 countries throughout the world concluded a three-year project in 1986 sponsored by the Fogarty International Center of the United States National Institutes of Health.[16] This group took a critical and comprehensive look at the state of antibiotic usage and antibiotic resistance worldwide. They found that current antibiotic production closely matched the needs of the world's population, that is, if all antibiotics were effective and resistance were not a deterrent. These conditions, however, are not present and the distribution of these antibiotics is highly unequal. In the developed world, antibiotics are plentiful. In areas of the world where they are sorely needed, antibiotics are available only in limited supply. Yet these are the areas with the highest frequency of infectious diseases. The reason for this hazardous health situation is poor public sanitation, particularly with regard to the water supply. To make matters worse, these are the same areas where antibiotic resistance poses the greatest threat to the population. Translated into public health parlance, this situation means more spread of disease and more resistance.

The Fogarty study also found that the frequency of resistance to some of the most common antibiotics had reached high levels among certain bacterial populations of individual countries where they appeared to persist. This finding meant that, although enough total antibiotics were being produced to cover the world, a good part of these antibiotics would not be useful in the face of large-scale resistance.

The levels of resistance varied by antibiotic and by country. The reasons for these differences were not clear, but could and should certainly take into account differences in patterns of antibiotic use, or differences in public health management. Studies addressing this point showed a vastly different country-to-country utilization of antibiotics and even variable administration in hospitals within the same country. For instance, in Japan, cephalosporin use per person was more than ten times that in Sweden and Australia and four to five times that in most other countries. To a great extent, this larger consumption in Japan was attributed to a financial gain received by the physician prescribing the cephalosporins. On the other hand, a financial incentive cannot explain the twofold difference found in the consumption of certain antibiotics in eight hospitals in Sweden.[17] That this kind of difference should exist in Sweden, where the diseases, the geography, and the people are so homogeneous, indicates that other factors are influencing decisions about antibiotic use. These differences must lie in the rationale behind the decisions of the physicians controlling the treatment. Understanding the reasons for different antibiotic utilization rates in Sweden and elsewhere would help to develop a plan to match antibiotic availability with a country's needs.

The Fogarty Task Force study found that, while frequency to resistance to particular antibiotics varied greatly with the microorganisms overall, distant countries still shared the same kinds of resistant strains of bacteria. Today, worldwide, about 30–50% of all *E. coli* commonly involved in urinary tract infections are resistant to penicillin drugs, tetracyclines, and other common antibiotics. In some areas almost 20% of the strains are resistant to trimethoprim-sulfamethoxazole (co-trimoxazole), the drug recommended as first choice for the treatment of urinary tract infections. Fortunately, we have other drugs on hand to treat these resistant infections, but the choices are decreasing. In parts of Asia, over 50% of *E. coli* are resistant to the fluoroquinolones.

A more diverse range of resistance frequencies is found for *Hemophilus influenzae*, which can cause ear infections, meningitis, and pneumonia. Here a resistance frequency range of 10–90% is noted to ampicillin, tetracyclines, and up to five different antibiotics, depending on the geographical location.

The Fogarty study further showed that each country of the world was dealing with the resistance problem at a somewhat different societal level. The more industrialized countries of North America and Europe were confronting diseases of resistant and multiresistant bacteria among individuals in particular communities or in hospitals. Most infectious diseases in the United States affect an individual or, at most, his or her family. On a rare occasion, larger groups have been infected, such as when epidemics of gastrointestinal diseases strike schools and nurseries. In the late 1980s, an epidemic of multiresistant *Shigella* causing diarrhea plagued two Indian reservations in the United States. Once again, alternative antibiotics and public health measures succeeded in curbing the outbreaks before they reached dangerous proportions. Unfortunately, this kind of successful outcome is not seen commonly in the developing world. Here, resistant bacteria often thwart treatment of large numbers of patients. The reason—inadequate public health measures to curb the spread of the infectious agents.

Although bearing lower numbers of people afflicted by infectious disease, the developed world has its own share of serious resistance problems. In the United States, for instance, the treatment of common community infections, such as ear infections, gonorrheal infections, and pneumonias, is gravely thwarted by resistance to penicillins and tetracyclines.

It was, in fact, the failure of antibiotics to treat common ear infections in children that launched the 1994 cover story in

Newsweek entitled "The End of Miracle Drugs?" This one event, more than any other, brought awareness in the United States and elsewhere of the antibiotic resistance problem as it confronts every household, in particular, our children.

Despite the unique and comprehensive participation and outcome of the Fogarty project, it had a sorrowful fate. Its aim to have an international congress devoted to the issue was denied, as was its plan for follow-up meetings to take control of what was seen by the eminent group as an escalating global problem. Political maneuverings and actions by pharmaceutical groups convinced U.S. officials and the National Institutes of Health, which sponsored the project, that the problem was being overstated and that support for the planned meeting and any future efforts should be withdrawn. Only a very condensed report reached publication. Many who worked on the project were alarmed, disappointed, and frustrated by such a unilateral decision. It is a sad commentary on the times. One can only wonder if this avant garde initiative had been allowed to continue with its mission, whether the global crisis of antibiotic resistance would be as grave as that which we face today.

International Response to Antibiotic Resistance: The Alliance for the Prudent Use of Antibiotics (APUA)

How does the world community deal with resistance on one hand and antibiotic availability on the other? The World Health Organization has convened many groups of experts to investigate the problem by identifying the factors causing resistance and finding the correct means of dealing with this issue. Their findings, recorded in a number of publications, emphasize that antibiotics are the primary selective agents for resistance and so their usage, whether too little or too much, must be evaluated and improved. Underlying these reports was the apparent need for national efforts to be carried out by local individuals working in concert with government authorities, to deal with the problem at the local level.

For many years, there existed no organized channel for communicating local situations to international audiences. Clearly there was a need for a consortium, an alliance of concerned people worldwide to deal with the issue from the grassroots level—from users and prescribers on up to heads of state. Such an organization arose as a result of a conference in the Dominican Republic in January 1981.

Over 200 participants from developing as well as developed countries convened in Santo Domingo to discuss the medical problems and ecology of resistance genes and their transferable vehicles—the plasmids. What emerged was a recognition that antibiotic resistance was not just the affliction of particular nations but a global problem. The meeting put aside taboos about talking about the problem; antibiotic resistance was worldwide and manifest in different ways in different countries. The overall message was clear—antibiotics were being misused, everywhere.

The participants recognized a need to publicize this message—to remove the constraints on talking about the problem and to inform people before it was really too late to take effective action. Only open discussion among nations could help control this mounting, now fully evident public health menace.

Out of this meeting came an "Antibiotic Misuse Statement" that was endorsed by hundreds of clinicians, researchers, and scientific societies worldwide. It declared, "We are faced with a worldwide public health problem," and went on to discuss antibiotic resistance and the major ways it was being propagated.

The statement was translated into many languages, including French, Spanish, Italian, Portuguese, Chinese, and Russian. It was formally presented at press conferences that took place simultaneously on August 4, 1981, in Boston, Massachusetts; Santo Domingo, Dominican Republic; Mexico City, Mexico; and São Paulo, Brazil (Figure 11.5).

The public responded with a flurry of questions and concern. To most, this was news—disconcerting news. *Newsweek* and *Time* magazines featured the statement and its message in their medical news of the week. Articles and editorials appeared in the *New York Times*, the *Washington Post* and newspapers throughout the world. The response was dramatic and, more importantly, international. The scientific journal *Nature* featured an entire page-long editorial entitled "Saving antibiotics from themselves." The statement of misuse served its initial purpose, to make the world aware of the gravity of the problem and its global presence.

The *Alliance for the Prudent Use of Antibiotics* (APUA) emerged from this meeting and its subsequent resolution. This internationally based group, whose present membership extends to more than 100 countries of the world, communicates basic tenets of proper antibiotic usage and the problems of antibiotic resistance to its members through a regular quarterly newsletter and various notices and forms of correspondence (Figure 11.6, page 308). It is the only organization of its kind dedicated solely to the improved use of and knowledge about a single therapeutic modality, not a disease. Its rationale is that antibiotics are crucial to all medical therapies involving people of all ages—in medicine, pediatrics, and surgery—and must be safeguarded vigilantly. Countries such as Bangladesh, Australia, China, Guatemala, and Venezuela formed groups or APUA chapters to deal with the issue locally. Currently there are 28 country-based chapters, with others in the planning stage. Through communication and education, the organization

Figure 11.5.   On August 4, 1981, pursuant to discussions about antibiotic misuse and resistance worldwide at a meeting in Santo Domingo, Dominican Republic, investigators in four cities worldwide presented an Antibiotic Misuse Statement. With the author (center; Dr. Levy) at this press conference in Boston were Dr. George Jacoby (left) of Harvard University Medical School and the Massachusetts General Hospital, and Nobel Laureate Dr. Walter Gilbert (right) of Harvard University (Photo Department, Tufts University School of Medicine).

seeks to promote improved use of antibiotics and to protect their long-term efficacy.

In order to be effective, APUA acts outside of political and economic pressures. Its members are individuals, doctors, dentists, pharmacists, veterinarians, biologists, microbiologists, public health officials, and others whose professions include handling antibiotics directly or confronting resistance in the home, hospital, or laboratory. This international group is making people all over the world cognizant of the resistance problem. It conveys the equally important message that antibiotic availability is important for disease eradication, not to be curtailed just when resistant variants appear. In many

Figure 11.6. The
Alliance for the Prudent
Use of Antibiotics
(www.apua.org), estab-
lished at the end of 1981,
has members from over
100 countries worldwide.
Through communication
and education, APUA ad-
vocates appropriate use of
antibiotics (APUA, Boston,
Massachusetts).

countries, this means making antibiotics *more* available, not
less available, while adhering to effective doses.

Communication and cooperation among all nations is necessary to win the battle against the looming problem of resistance. Although one country can maintain strict adherence to
better policies of antibiotic use, it would still run the risk of
picking up and propagating resistant strains from other countries that are not so diligent. Through prudent usage, a resistant pathogen arising in one country could be contained in
the country of origin and successfully eliminated before it had
the chance to spread to the rest of the world. Everyone concerned will admit that it is a slow process, but giant steps do
occur, such as the removal of fixed combinations of antibiotics
in Spain, removal of over-the-counter sale of antibiotics in

Chile, and the greatly improved antibiotic usage in Australia and Brazil. What each country needs is support from its government in order to establish an antibiotic policy, an achievable reality in the wake of a global effort.

The findings of the Fogarty study more than a decade ago are just as relevant today, except that the situation is worse. We have more than enough antibiotics to go around, but the distribution is unequal. Misuse continues in all areas where antibiotics are being applied. Resistance frequencies have increased. Over the past decade, other reports have joined Fogarty in asking for global attention to this international problem. In particular, in 2001 the World Health Organization released its "Global Strategy for Containment of Antimicrobial Resistance." The APUA produced its summation of 25 documents over the past 15 years dealing with advice from experts on antibiotic use and resistance, which accompanied the WHO report. The fact that so many documents existed attests to the attention paid by experts to the problem, but little action followed to resolve it. The American College of Physicians–American Society of Internal Medicine produced nine back-to-back publications in the *Annals of Internal Medicine* that advised physicians on how to best use antibiotics for upper respiratory tract infections in order to curtail resistance.

The esteemed House of Lords in the United Kingdom convened a subgroup of its Science and Technology Committee in 1998, headed by Lord Soulsby of Swaltham, to evaluate antibiotic resistance. Their superbly written document highlights the problems of resistance as it faces the United Kingdom and the world at large. It joins others in relating the problem of resistance and urges legislative action, seeking support to curtail this international problem.

Their report estimated that one-third of prescriptions from physicians to patients was not needed. They recommended major re-education of doctors and consumers, in particular mothers who pressured their physicians to prescribe drugs for their children. Lord Soulsby stated, "Misuse and overuse of antibiotics are now threatening to undermine all the early promises and success in curing disease. But the greatest threat is complacency from ministers, the medical profession, the veterinary services, the farming community, and the public at large. Action must start now if we are not to return to the bad old days of incurable diseases before antibiotics were available."

All reports stress that one country cannot dictate to another country how to distribute or control the use of antibiotics, but a general plan could be derived to help stem the tide of antibiotic resistance. This growing problem requires a universal effort, with all countries working together toward a common goal, similar to recent world forums on global warming and fishing rights. At a minimum, certain guidelines can be drawn based on current scientific information. These guidelines can focus on antibiotic use and the existence of resistance. The kinds of bacteria causing the most common diseases should be identified in each country. Their susceptibility to antibiotics should be made well known. Then, appropriate antibiotics can be purchased, distributed, and used effectively in that particular country. It is important to remember, however, that every country is connected through the microbial network. The antibiotic needs of each country should be met, but cautious and discriminate use must be practiced everywhere since every human being's health is at stake. Otherwise, the single country's efforts will be fraught with failure as new forms of resistant microorganisms travel across national and international borders.

Many organizations are now aligned to reverse the problem of resistance by taking a major stand on the important factor promoting that resistance—the misuse of antibiotics.

Goals for the Future

It is inappropriate to point a finger at any one particular participant using or dispensing antibiotics as the cause of the resistance problem. As noted earlier, antibiotic use is pervasive in our society. In each phase of antibiotic production, prescription, and use, there are some people who act responsibly and some who do not. An understanding must be reached in each area in order to see that inappropriate usage is curtailed. When incorrect use or faulty prescriptions persist despite medical and public opinion, actions should be taken to deal vigorously with the offenders. This response, as we mentioned before, can come directly only from local medical authorities. The most effective group, in the United States at least, is the prepay medical systems that monitor both patient use and physician prescribing profiles. If users and prescribers agree to look at their usage patterns more carefully, then industry members should also ascribe importance to seeing that their products are used rationally and effectively. The economics of the issue cannot be brushed aside, but then, there is no evidence that good and ethical practices will bring lower profits.

The goal in the next decade is to make antibiotics more available in the areas where they are most needed and to discourage frivolous use in areas where they are currently being overused. Education must remove the false impressions and attitudes about these drugs in the minds of the consumer and the prescriber. All concerned groups should carefully examine the factors that cause the emergence of resistance and help curtail these resistant strains as they appear in one country or another. It is efforts such as those displayed by the Fogarty International Center, the World Health Organization, and the *Alliance for the Prudent Use of Antibiotics* that are bringing global attention to the fact that resistant bacteria are a continuing problem. It is these and other groups yet to be formed who may help conquer this impending threat. But they need the support of the world population—consumers and prescribers alike.

Faced with the realization that the societal effect of antibiotics makes them a special class of therapeutics, I suggest that they be given a separate status and drug category through the federal regulatory agencies. After all, the individual use and misuse of an antibiotic are of consequence not only to the individual but also to society at large, especially as misuse events increase. No other drugs have this effect. Provider and consumer should realize that antibiotics are special, not to be regarded like any other drugs such as analgesics, heart or kidney medications, or endocrine replacement therapies. If they can be given a special category, then unique considerations can be applied to them, such as prolonged patent life and tax benefits to pharmaceutical companies in exchange for monitoring antibiotic resistance and marketing strategies that will curtail the emergence of resistance. A special category for antibiotics will help bring attention to their unique societal feature—the effect on the environment of microbes shared by members of all society, locally and throughout the world.

The resistance gene pool is constantly multiplying, as are the numbers of microorganisms resistant to more than one antibiotic. If we ignore the problem, single-drug therapy will simply become obsolete. Our goal should be to attempt to maintain the efficacy of the antibiotics we have by determining which diseases they can still eradicate and which microorganisms are still largely susceptible (Figure 11.7). Studies that reveal the basis for resistance should be encouraged and supported. These could lead to the rational design of new drugs or special drug treatments that are not subject to the resistance mechanism. Once developed, we should use the new antibiotics appropriately.

The antibiotic myth continues in far too many households and minds of people worldwide. On a more optimistic note,

Figure 11.7. Mankind wins the next round. Through concerted efforts on the part of everyone developing, dispensing, and consuming antibiotics, humans can emerge victorious in their struggles with the infectious microbes (Herbert Hächler, University of Zurich, Zurich, Switzerland).

never before have so many organizations worldwide agreed that resistance is a major public health problem that needs to be addressed. The World Health Organization named it one of the three major health problems of the new century. Organizations representing different disciplines, from dermatologists to dentists to ophthalmologists to microbiologists, are dealing with the question of how best to confront and curtail the spread of antibiotic-resistant bacteria. This is a far cry from the situation in the beginning of the last decade, at the time this book was first written. Complacency reigned then, and ignorance and denial were prominent. We can look forward to a more knowledgeable public in the 21st century, but the crisis we are living through now could well become a disaster if proper use of antibiotics is not entertained widely and new drugs are not made available for the care of our patients suffering from resistant infections.

At the same time, we should put into action a new public-awareness model for the use of antibiotics that will protect the new drugs from becoming rapidly outdated through the same resistance problems. This kind of commitment should move us toward using antibiotics more wisely, more efficiently, and more appropriately. We could then control the rise in antibiotic resistance and assure the success of antibiotics now and for generations to come.

Epilogue

Anthrax, Bioterrorism, and Antibiotic Stockpiling: Consequences Beyond the Scare

Last month, following on the heels of the September 11, 2001, attack on the World Trade Center and Pentagon, U.S. citizens were, for the first time, confronted with the reality of a bioterrorism agent—anthrax. A national public health crisis rapidly emerged, not only because of anthrax, but also because of its impact on antibiotic use.

Microscopic "spores" of a potentially deadly bacterium, *Bacillus anthracis*, were transmitted in letters, first to a publishing house, then to members of Congress and the television networks. In response to media reports, the public sought antibiotics on an unprecedented scale. Citizens without risk of the disease began stockpiling antibiotics as a safeguard against a future potential event. Clearly, under these conditions, control of antibiotic misuse is not possible, and an accelerated propagation of resistant bacteria becomes a looming reality. If any event threatens to epitomize the "antibiotic paradox", the reaction of the American people to the possibility of widespread anthrax in the fall of 2001 certainly does. An experiment in microbial evolution has been launched.

The anthrax bacillus, which gets its name from the Greek word for "coal" because it produces a "coal-black" skin infection, can exist in two forms. One is multiplying and able to form colonies on agar plates. The second is a resting or protective "spore" state, during which the organism can survive for long periods despite extremes of temperature. The inhalation of five to ten thousand spores can result in airborne pulmonary anthrax, the most severe form of disease.

Once in the lungs, the spores sprout the actively multiplying bacteria which produce toxins, leading to a hemorrhagic disease and fluid accumulation. Death comes to four out of five people infected, if not treated early. Another route of anthrax infection is through a break in the skin. Fortunately in these patients, disease is limited and obvious, and treatment can begin before it becomes more generalized and fatal. The third route of infection is uncommon—via ingestion of spores or organisms leading to gastrointestinal disease.

Bacillus anthracis is a common bacterium found in soils and among animals. In France, the areas of buried remains of animals in the Savoie and Normandy are natural havens for the organism. Local dwellers used to call them "champs maudits" (or "cursed fields") because of the fear attached to the illness. In the United States, the bacteria are found associated with wild and domesticated animals with often no evidence of disease. Any trained microbiologist can isolate and grow the organism. It is the harvesting and developing of anthrax into a biologic weapon which requires additional technical skill. For successful bioterrorism, the individual spores must not stick to each other as they do in nature. As single spores, they remain airborne longer and able to get through the nasal passages and into the lung. Additives can be used to keep the spores apart, but if they cause a cough, the spores will be expelled. Consequently, a non-irritating, fine powder must be selected for this purpose. Thus, there is a certain precision involved in preparing the spores for bioterrorism.

When anthrax was first identified as a biowarfare agent in the United States, the Food & Drug Administration and the Centers for Disease Control and Prevention recommended ciprofloxacin, an antibiotic sold under the name *Cipro* by the Bayer Pharmaceutical Company in Germany for treatment and prophylaxis. Ciprofloxacin is a member of the fluoroquinolone group of broad-spectrum antibiotics that have been life-saving for many critically ill patients since their introduction some 14 years ago. *Cipro* was first chosen for anthrax because the susceptibility of the bacteria to antibiotics was unknown and it was a "best guess" that resistance was unlikely. Later, when the organism was found susceptible to many different antibiotics, a tetracycline, namely, doxycycline, and a penicillin, (Penicillin G), were also approved. Other antibiotics were recently added to the effective list. The current recommendation of 60 days for treatment and prophylaxis—far longer than most antibiotic regimens—arose from studies in monkeys which showed recurrence of disease after 30 days of antibiotic therapy. For the inhalation form of the disease, therapy must be started at the first signs of illness, which resemble features of the flu, namely fever, malaise, and lower respiratory discomfort. Usually more than one antibiotic is provided because of the severity of the disease and possibility of resistance.

During the 1950s, my father, a practicing physician in Wilmington, DE, found cutaneous anthrax among workers at a local leather factory. In those days, penicillins or tetracyclines were the treatment of choice; resistance was not an issue. Fortunately to date, no isolate anywhere has been found resistant. However, concern about resistance arises from the knowledge that the USSR's now-discontinued biologic warfare program had engineered penicillin resistance into the anthrax bacillus, making this a much more formidable weapon. Introducing resistance to other antibiotics is not difficult and lies within the technical expertise of many microbiology students. Individual genes for resistance to penicillin and tetracyclines are readily available as we discussed elsewhere in this book. Resistance to fluoroquinolones requires at least two mutations in the chromosomal gene which codes for the target protein for the drug. While feasible, the necessity of more than one mutation does make it more difficult to acquire resistance to this family of antibiotics.

As the news of anthrax spread, almost overnight *Cipro* became an everyday household word. Residents in areas of New York, Washington and Florida, where anthrax was first discovered, as well as many other parts of the United States, began seeking *Cipro* for themselves as protection against a full-fledged attack. Individual demand and overprescription by physicians caused a run on pharmacies for ciprofloxacin, leaving some pharmacies depleted of the drug. Prescriptions were filled and sent by express mail from web sites. One individual reported buying and receiving six pills, a three-day supply, with the approval for 19 refills! In a relatively short period of time, bottles of a powerful antibiotic were put into the hands of people to be used "just in case". By the end of October, an ABC News/Washington Post poll estimated that 2% of Americans had acquired the drug. That estimate translates to millions of people who have stockpiled ciprofloxacin. Since the initial symptoms of anthrax resemble a viral illness, how does anyone know when to use the medication? Consumption would likely begin at the first respiratory symptoms. Given the already documented overuse of antibiotics by consumers for the common cold, it is expected that the bottle of *Cipro*, originally purchased for protection against anthrax, might be used for any cold or flu symptoms. This possibility is even greater since the anthrax scare has occurred as the U.S. greets the cold and flu season.

There is no control over how the consumer will respect an acquired antibiotic. A 60-day supply is far more than any antibiotic stockpiles I have ever seen in medicine cabinets. The run on *Cipro* thus becomes a further threat to our national health and welfare. Ingestion of this drug by the millions of people who stockpiled it will cause a significant change in the microbial environment. The currently small numbers of resistant, disease-causing bacteria, such as the pneumococcus, the gonococcus, *E.coli*, and *Pseudomonas*, will, under the pressure of massive antibiotic selection, increase in numbers and eventually become the cause of hard-to-treat infections. Today, by one estimate, there are two U.S. hospital deaths each hour associated with a resistant bacterial infection. There could be far more disease problems (and even deaths) arising from resistance due to the misuse of ciprofloxacin than will be incurred from people affected by anthrax. Only time will tell.

No one is proposing that the prophylactic use of antibiotics not be provided for those directly exposed to anthrax, or for anyone in the same vicinity where anthrax spores have been detected. This use is rational and indicated—a necessary protection against possible death. Exposed individuals can be treated prophylacticly with one of several antibiotics currently approved. Having a choice of antibiotic is important because it avoids single drug use by large numbers of the same community, which speeds up the selection of strains resistant to the drug.

Not since the discovery of penicillin has an antibiotic attained the notoriety of worldwide, front-page news—a phenomenon that the media dubbed "Cipromania". The stockpiling of *Cipro*, or any other antibiotic in response to an incipient bioterrorism event, permits self-medication at its worst. The risk posed by the extensive use of these stockpiled drugs is an accelerated evolution of resistant bacteria that has never been witnessed before. Moreover, although side effects from these antibiotics may affect only a few percent of those taking them, the numbers of such patients seeking medical advice will increase significantly.

There have been deaths from the anthrax attack, but fortunately other infected persons were cured with antibiotics. As one astute Parisian physician said, "Les antibiotiques sont, quand-même, nec-essaires" (Antibiotics are, after all, still necessary.) And for anthrax, they can make the difference between life and death. As with any disease, however, we must reserve their use for those in true need.

Anthrax is not the only biowarfare disease. To be successful, biowarfare agents must be readily harvested and prepared for delivery, in a controllable way, and be easily spread with a high rate of killing. Other potential bacterial agents include *Yersinia pestis* (the cause of plague) and *Franciscella tularensis* causing tularemia, a systemic, potentially fatal disease that can be naturally contracted by insect bites, drinking contaminated water, or breathing contaminated air. In Oklahoma, in the year 2000, seven people were hospitalized with tularemia in a two-week period. In the spring of 2001, several patients contracted tularemia on Martha's Vineyard. In both instances, authorities were on the alert for a possible terrorist act. Fortunately, neither suspicion proved true, and the patients recovered under antibiotic treatment.

A host of viruses, including those for small pox and for the different hemorrhagic fevers, e.g. Ebola, Marburg, and Lassa, are other potential agents. Also, toxins produced by bacteria, such as *Clostridium botulinum* and *Clostridium perfringens*, can cause fatal disease when ingested. Neither toxins nor viruses can be treated by antibiotics, and would have to be controlled, if possible, by vaccines. Unfortunately, few antivirals are available. For that reason, the small pox vaccination program has been recently stepped up.

The approach to all bacterial biowarfare agents should be rational use of antibiotics for prophylaxis and treatment. Physicians, public health authorities, and fellow citizens should emphatically discourage individual stockpiling of these drugs. The alternative outcome, as presented by the current anthrax scare, is massive stockpiling and self-medication with a potentially significant impact on the treatment of other disease-causing bacteria. Public health officials must aggressively manage the crisis and citizens must follow their directives. All of us need to be aware of the dangers and consequences of antibiotic overuse —namely, the emergence of bacteria no longer treatable with these life-saving therapeutics.

STUART B. LEVY, MD
Boston, Massachusetts
November 2001

References Cited

Chapter One

1. The *Boston Herald*, November 29, 1942.
2. The *Boston Sunday Globe*, November 29, 1942.
3. The *Boston Daily Globe*, November 30, 1942.
4. The *Boston Daily Globe*, December 2, 1942.
5. The *New York Times*, p. 21, June 26, 1945.

Chapter Two

1. Tiberio, V. Sugli estratti di alcune muffe Annali di Igiene Sperimentale 5:91–103, 1895
2. Waksman, S. A. The microbiology of soil and the antibiotics. In: *The Impact of the Antibiotics on Medicine and Society*. (Galdston, I., Ed.). International Universities Press, Inc. New York, p. 3, 1958.
3. Cowen, D. L. and Segelman, A. B. *Antibiotics in Historical Perspective*. Merck Sharp and Dohme International, Rahway, NJ, 1981.

Chapter Three

1. Ebbell, B. *The Papyrus Ebers*. Lewin and Munksgaard, Copenhagen, 1937.
2. Contenau, G. *La Médicine en Assyrie et en Babylone*. Librairie Maloine, Paris, 1938.
3. Walsh, J. J. *The Popes and Science*. Fordham University Press, New York. Appendix III (translation provided in *J. Amer. Med. Assoc.*, January 1908), pp. 419–423, 1911.

4. Guerra, F. *American Medical Bibliography 1639–1783*. Lathrop C. Harper Inc., New York, 1962.
5. Theobald, J. *Every Man His Own Physician*, Third Edition. London, 1764.

Chapter Four

1. Lenski, R. E., Simpson, S. C., Nguyen, T. T. Genetic analysis of a plasmid-encoded, host genotype-specific enhancement of bacterial fitness. *J. Bacteriol* 176:3140–3147, 1994.
2. Hall, R. M. and Collins, C. M. Mobile gene cassettes and integrons: capture and spread of genes by site-specific recombination. *Mol. Microbiology* 15:593–600, 1995.

Chapter Five

1. Cohen, D., Creek, G., and Sayers, R. *Haemophilus influenzae* infections in American children living in the U.K. *Lancet i:*101, 1982.

Chapter Six

1. Bates, J., Jordens, J. Z., and Griffiths, D. T. Farm animals as a putative reservoir for vancomycin resistant enterococcal infections in man. *J. Antimicrob. Chemother.* 34: 507–514, 1994.
2. Report of WHO Meeting on the medical impact of the use of antimicrobial drugs in food animals, 1997.
3. Pritchard, W. R. and Loew, F. M. Veterinary Medicine: Looking toward the 21st century. In: *Perspectives on the Health Professions*. Chapter 1. (O'Neil, E. H., Ed.). Pew Health Professions Programs, Duke University, 1990.

Chapter Nine

1. *La Revue Prescrire*, p. 2, April 1984.
2. Hook, E. H., Brady, W. E., Reichart, C. A. *et al.* Determinants of emergence of antibiotic-resistant *Neisseria gonorrhoeae*. *J. Infect. Dis.* 159:900–907, 1989.
3. Nelson, W. L., Kennedy, D. L., Lao, C. S., and Kuritsky, J. N. Outpatient systemic antiinfective use by children in the United States, 1977–1986. *Pediat. Infect. Dis. J.* 7:505–509, 1988.

4. Reves, R. R., Fong, M., Pickering, L. K. *et al*. Risk factors for fecal colonization with trimethoprim-resistant and multiresistant *Escherichia coli* among children in day-care centers in Houston, Texas. *Antimicrob. Agents Chemother. 34*:1429–1434, 1990.

5. Corpet, D. E. Antibiotic resistance from food. *N. Engl. J. Med. 318*:1206–1207, 1988.

6. Wang, F. and Tai, T-Y. People's Republic of China: clinical antibiotic use. *APUA Newsletter 4*:4:1, 7, 1986.

Chapter Eleven

1. Welch, H. Antibiotics 1943–1955: Their development and role in present-day society. In: *The Impact of Antibiotics on Medicine and Society* (Galdston, I., Ed.). International Universities Press, Inc. New York, p. 85, 1958.

2. Levy, S. B. Starting life resistance-free. *N. Engl. J. Med. 323*:335–337, 1990.

3. Miller, Y. W., Eady, E. A., Lacey, R. W., *et al*. Sequential antibiotic therapy for acne promotes the carriage of resistant staphylococci on the skin of contacts. *J. Antimicrob. Chemother 38*: 829–37, 1996.

4. Lester, S. C., del Pilar Pla, M., Wang, F. *et al*. The carriage of *Escherichia coli* resistant to antimicrobial agents by healthy children in Boston, in Caracas, Venezuela and in Qin Pu, China. *N. Engl. J. Med. 323*:285–289, 1990.

5. Levy, S. B. Antibiotic resistance: an ecological imbalance. In *Antibiotic resistance: origins, evolution, selection and spread*. (Chadwick, D. J. and Goode, J., Eds.) Wiley, Chichester, London (Ciba Foundation Symposium 207), pp. 1–14, 1997.

6. Montefiore, D. G., Rotimi, V. O., and Adeyeme-Doro, O. Antibiotic resistance in Nigeria: impact on drug choice. *APUA Newsletter 9*:2:1, 6–8, 1991.

7. Lee, D. Changing antibiotic utilization patterns in Costa Rica. *APUA Newsletter 9*:1:7–8, 1991.

8. Macauley, C. Antibiotic usage in an outpatient clinic—Thailand 1984. *APUA Newsletter 3*:4:4–5, 1985.

9. Bennish, M. Increasing resistance among *Shigella* isolates in Bangladesh: will a rational use drug policy help? *APUA Newsletter 9*:4:6–7, 1991.

10. Azof, A., Solter, S. Mizan, M., and Hamed, A. F. Antibiotic use; Aceh Province, Indonesia. *APUA Newsletter 4*:3:1,6, 1986.

11. Summers, A. O., Vimy, M., and Lorscheider, F. "Silver" dental fillings provoke an increase in mercury and antibiotic resistant bacteria in the mouth and intestines of primates. *APUA Newsletter* 9:3:4–5, 1991.

12. Holmberg, S. D., Solomon, S. L. and Blake, P. A. Health and economic impacts of antimicrobial resistance. *Rev. Infect. Dis.* 9:1065–1078, 1987.

13. Phelps, C. E. Bug/Drug Resistance. *Medical Care* 27:194–203, 1989.

14. Rubin, R., Harrington, C. A., Poon, A., *et al.* The economic impact of *Staphylococcus aureus* infection in New York City hospitals. *Emerg. Infect. Dis.* 5:9–17, 1999.

15. Swartz *et al.* Human health risks with the subtherapeutic use of penicillins or tetracyclines in animal feed. National Academy Press, Washington, D.C., p. 194, 1989.

16. Levy, S. B., Burke, J., and Wallace, E. (Eds.). Antibiotic use and antibiotic resistance worldwide. *Rev. Infect. Dis.* 9:Suppl 3, 1987.

17. Jansson, C., and Skold, O. Variations on the use of antibiotics among Swedish hospitals. *APUA Newsletter* 8:1:2–3, 1990.

Bibliography

Chapter 1

Cope, O. Care of the victims of the Cocoanut Grove fire at the Massachusetts General Hospital. *N. Engl. J. Med. 229*:138–147, 1943.

Hobby, G. L. *Penicillin Meeting the Challenge.* Yale University Press, New Haven, 1989.

Macionis, J. Boston's nightclub tragedy (1942). *Inferno*, pp. 147–163, 1967.

Sheehan, J., and Ross, R. N. The fire that made penicillin famous. *Yankee Magazine*, pp. 125–203, 1982.

Chapter 2

Abraham, E. P., Chain, E., Fletcher, C. M. *et al.* Further observations on penicillin. *The Lancet*, pp. 177–188, August 16, 1941.

Chain, E., Florey, H. W., Gardner, A. D. *et al.* Penicillin as a chemotherapeutic agent. *The Lancet*, pp. 226–228, August 24, 1940.

Fleming, A. On the antibacterial action of cultures of a *Penicillium*, with special reference to their use in the isolation of *B. influenzae. Brit. J. Exp. Path. 10*:226–236, 1929.

Fleming, A. (Ed.). *Penicillin: Its Practical Application.* Butterworths and Co. Ltd., London, 1946.

Florey, H. W. The use of micro-organisms for therapeutic purposes. *Brit. Med. J.*, pp. 635–642, November 10, 1945.

Gray, G. W. Antibiosis. *Scientific American*, pp. 27–34, August, 1944.

Life magazine, pp. 58–59, July 17, 1944.

MacFarlane, G. *Alexander Fleming. The Man and the Myth.* Harvard University Press, Cambridge, 1984.

Moburg, C. L., and Cohn, Z. A. (Eds.). *Launching the Antibiotic Era.* The Rockefeller University Press, New York, 1990.

Pasteur, L. La theorie des germes et ses applications à la medecine et à la chirugie. Oeuvres de Pasteur. *C. R. Acad. Sci.* LXXXVI, April 29, 1878.

Sedillot, C. De l'influence des decouvertes de M. Pasteur sur les progres de la chirugie. *C. R. Acad. Sci.* LXXXVI, p. 634–640, 1878.

Time magazine, pp. 61–68, May 15, 1944.

Vuillemin, P. Antibiose et symbiose. *C. R. Assoc. Fr. Acad. Sci.* 2:525–543. Seance du 14 aout, 1889.

Chapter 3

Bryan, C. P. *The Papyrus Ebers.* Geoffrey Blis, London, 1930.

Buchan, W. *Domestic Medicine or the Family Physician.* Royal College of Physicians, Edinburgh, 2nd American edition, Philadelphia, 1774.

Garrison, F. H. *Introduction to the History of Medicine.* 4th edition. W. B. Saunders, Philadelphia, 1929.

Gordon, B. L. *Medicine Throughout Antiquity.* F. A. Davis Co., Philadelphia, 1949.

Guthrie, D. *A History of Medicine.* Thomas Nelson and Sons Ltd., New York, 1945.

Inglis, B. *A History of Medicine.* World Publishing Company, Cleveland, 1965.

Majno, G. *The Healing Hand: Man and Wound in the Ancient World.* Harvard University Press, Cambridge, MA, 1975.

Moir, D. M. *Outlines of the Ancient History of Medicine.* William Blakewood, Edinburgh, 1831.

Netter, W., transl. of Peters, H. *Pictorial History of Ancient Pharmacy and Medicine.* Engelhard & Co., Chicago, 1889.

Chapter 4

Chadwick, D. J., and Goode, J. (Eds.). *Antibiotic resistance: origins, evolution, selection, and spread.* (CIBA Foundation Symposium 207). John Wiley and Sons, 1997.

Chow, J. W., Fine, M. J., and Shlaes, D. M. *Enterobacter* bacteremia: clinical features and emergence of antibiotic resistance during therapy. *Ann. Int. Med.* 115:585–590, 1991.

Croft, B. A. Arthropod resistance to insecticides: a key to pest control failures and successes in North American apple orchards. *Ent. Exp. Appl.* 31:88–110, 1982.

Datta, N., Faiers, M. C., Reeves, D. S. *et al.* R factors in *Escherichia coli* in faeces after oral chemotherapy in general practice. *The Lancet ii:* 312–315, 1971.

Davis, C. D., and Anandan, J. The evolution of R factor: a study of a "pre-antibiotic" community in Borneo. *N. Engl. J. Med.* 282:117–122, 1970.

Gardner, P., Smith, D. H., Beer, H., and Moellering, R. C., Jr. Recovery of resistance (R) factors from a drug-free community. *The Lancet*, pp. 774–776, October 11, 1969.

George, A. M. and Levy, S. B. Amplifiable resistance to tetracycline, chloramphenicol, and other antibiotics in *Escherichia coli:* identification of a non-plasmid mediated efflux system for tetracycline. *J. Bacteriol.* 155:531–540, 1983.

Harrison, P. F., and Lederberg, J. (Eds.). Antimicrobial resistance: issues and options. Institute of Medicine, National Academy of Sciences, 1998.

Heath, P. T., Booy, R., Azzopardi, H. J. *et al.* Non-type b *Haemophilus influenzae* disease: clinical and epidemiologic characteristics in the *Haemophilus influenzae* type b vaccine era. *Pediat. Infect. Dis.* 20:300–305, 2001.

Hiramatsu, K. Vancomycin resistance in staphylococci. *Drug Res. Updates* 1:135–150, 1998.

Hughes, V. M., and Datta, N. Conjugative plasmids in bacteria of the "pre-antibiotic" era. *Nature 302*:725–726, 1983.

Kloos, W. E. Effect of single antibiotic therapy on *Staphylococcus* community structure. *APUA Newsletter 5*:4:1–2, 1987.

Levy, S. B. The challenge of antibiotic resistance. *Scientific American 278*:46–53, 1998.

Levy, S. B., and Miller, R. V. (Eds.). *Gene Transfer in the Environment.* McGraw-Hill Publishing Co., New York, 1989.

Levy, S. B., Marshall, B., Schluederberg, S. *et al.* High frequency of antimicrobial resistance in human fecal flora. *Antimicrob. Agents Chemother. 32*:1801–1806, 1988.

Mare, I. J. Incidence of R factors among gram-negative bacteria in drug-free human and animal communities. *Nature* (London) *220*:1046–1047, 1968.

Mare, I. J., and Coetzee, J. N. The incidence of transmissible drug resistance factors among strains of *Escherichia coli* in the Pretoria area. *S.A. Med. J.*, pp. 980–981, November 5, 1966.

Moller, J. K., Bak, A. L., Stenderup, A., Zachariae, H., and Afzelius, H. Changing patterns of plasmid-mediated resistance during tetracycline therapy. *Antimicrob. Agents Chemother. 11*:388–391, 1977.

Murray, B. E., Renismer, E. R., and DuPont, H. L. Emergence of high-level trimethoprim resistance in fecal *Escherichia coli* during oral administration of trimethoprim or trimethoprim-sulfamethoxazole. *N. Engl. J. Med.* 306:130–135, 1982.

Novick, R. P. Penicillinase plasmids of *Staphylococcus aureus. Fed. Proc.* 27:29–38, 1967.

O'Brien, T. F., del Pilar Pla, M., Mayer, K. H. *et al.* Intercontinental spread of a new antibiotic resistance gene on an epidemic plasmid. *Science* 230:87–88, 1985.

Roberts, M. C. Tetracycline resistance determinants: mechanisms of action, regulation of expression, genetic mobility, and distribution. *FEMS Microb. Review.* 19:1–24. 1996.

Rolland, R. M., Hausfater, G., Marshall, B., and Levy, S. B. Antibiotic-resistant bacteria in wild primates: Increased prevalence in baboons feeding on human refuse. *Appl. Env. Microbiol.* 49:791–794, 1985.

Sanders, C. C. New ß-lactams: new problems for the internist. *Ann. Int. Med.* 115:650–651, 1991.

Smith, D. H. Salmonella with transferable drug resistance. *N. Engl. J. Med.* 275:625–630, 1966.

Sugarman, B., and Pesanti, E. Treatment failures secondary to *in vivo* development of drug resistance by microorganisms. *Rev. Infect. Dis.* 2:153–167, 1980.

Tauxe, R. V., Cavanagh, T. R., and Cohen, M. L. Interspecies gene transfer *in vivo* producing an outbreak of multiply resistant Shigellosis. *J. Infect. Dis.* 160:1067–1070, 1989.

Zscheck, K. K., Hull, R., and Murray, B. E. Restriction mapping and hybridization studies of a ß-lactamase-encoding fragment from *Streptococcus (Enterococcus) faecalis. Antimicrob. Agents Chemother.* 32:768–769, 1988.

Chapter 5

Broome, C. V., Mortimer, E. A., Katz, S. L. *et al.* Use of chemoprophylaxis to prevent the spread of *Hemophilus influenzae* b in day-care facilities. *N. Engl. J. Med.* 316:1226–1228, 1987.

Col, N. F., and O'Connor, R. W. Estimating worldwide current antibiotic usage: Report of Task Force 1. *Rev. Infect. Dis.* 9:S232–243, 1987.

Knapp, J. S., Zenilman, J. M., Biddle, J. W. *et al.* Distribution and frequency of strains of *Neisseria gonorrhoeae* with plasmid-mediated, high-level resistance to tetracycline (TRNG) in the United States. *J. Infect. Dis.* 155:819–822, 1987.

Kunin, C. M., Lipton, H. L., Tupasi, T. *et al.* Social, behavioral and practical factors affecting antibiotic use worldwide: report of Task Force 4. *Rev. Infect. Dis. 9*:S270–285, 1987.

Parker, C. W. Drug Allergy. *N. Engl. J. Med. 292*:732–736, 1975.

Pichichero, M. E. (Ed.) Judicious use of antibiotics in pediatric respiratory infections 2000. *Pediat. Infect. Des. 19*:909–943, 2000.

Polk, H. C. Jr., and Christmas, A. B. Prophylactic antibiotics in surgery and surgical wound infections. *Amer. Surg. 66*:105–111, 2000.

Reid, G., and Sobel, J. D. Bacterial adherence in the pathogenesis of urinary tract infection: a review. *Rev. Infect. Dis. 9*:470–487, 1987.

Seppala, H., Klaukka, T., Vuopio-Varkila, J. *et al.* The effect of changes in the consumption of macrolide antibiotics on erythromycin resistance in group A streptococci in Finland. *New Eng. J. Med.* 337:441–6, 1997.

Seppala, H., Nissinen, A., Jarvinen, H. *et al.* Resistance to erythromycin in Group A streptococci. *N. Engl. J. Med. 326*:292–297, 1992.

Takata, G. S., Chan, L. S., Shekelle, P. *et al.* Evidence assessment of management of acute otitis media: The role of antibiotics in treatment of uncomplicated acute otitis media. *Pediatrics 108*:239–247, 2001.

Chapter 6

Anderson, E. S., and Lewis, M. J. Characterization of a transfer factor associated with drug resistance in *Salmonella typhimurium*. *Nature 208*:843–849, 1965.

Edel, W., Van Schothorsat, M., Van Leusden, F. M., and Kampelmacher, E. H. Epidemiological studies on *Salmonella* in a certain area. *Zbl. Bakt Hyg. I. Abt. Orig. A 242*:468–480, 1978.

Holmberg, S. D. *et al.* Drug resistant *Salmonella* from animals fed antibiotics. *N. Engl. J. Med. 311*:617–622, 1987.

Hummel, R., Tschape, H., and Witte, W. Spread of plasmid-mediated nourseothricin resistance in connection with antibiotic use in animal husbandry. *J. Basic Microb. 26*:461–466, 1986.

Levy, S. B. Antibiotic use for growth promotion in animals: ecologic and public health consequences. *J. Food Protection 50*:616–620, 1987.

Levy, S. B. Multidrug resistance: a sign of the times. *New Eng. J. Med. 338*:1376–1378, 1998.

Levy, S. B., Fitzgerald, G. G., and Macone, A. B. Changes in the intestinal flora of farm personnel after introduction of tetracycline-supplemented feed on a farm. *N. Engl. J. Med. 295*:583–588, 1976.

Lyons, R. W., Samples, C. L., DeSilva, H. N. *et al.* An epidemic of resistant *Salmonella* in a nursery: animal-to-animal spread. *J. Amer. Med. Assoc.* 243:546–547, 1980.

Marshall, B. M., Petrowski, D., and Levy, S. B. Inter and intraspecies spread of *E. coli* in a farm environment in the absence of antibiotic usage. *Proc. Nat'l Acad. Sci.* (USA) 87:6609–6613, 1990.

Mellon, M., Berbrook, C, and Benbrook, K. L. *Hogging It.* Union of Concerned Scientists, 2001.

Pivnick, H., Blanchard, B. and D'Aoust, I. J. Prevention of Salmonella infection in chicks by treatment with fecal cultures from mature chickens (Nurmi cultures). *J. Food Protection* 44:909–916, 1981.

Riley, L. W. *et al.* Evaluation of isolated cases of salmonellosis by plasmid profile analysis: introduction and transmission of a bacterial clone by precooked roast beef. *J. Infect. Dis.* 148:12–17, 1983.

Riley, L. W. *et al.* Importance of host factors in human salmonella caused by multiresistant strains of *Salmonella. J. Infect. Dis.* 149:878–883, 1984.

Rolland, R., Hausfater, G., Marshall, B. and Levy, S. B. Increased frequency of antibiotic resistant gut flora in wild baboons in contact with human refuse. *Appl. Environ. Microbiol.* 49:791–794, 1985.

Ryan, C. A., Nickels, M. K. *et al.* Massive outbreak of antimicrobial-resistant salmonellosis traced to pasteurized milk. *J. Amer. Med. Assoc.* 258:3269–3279, 1987.

Schifferli, D. M., and Beachey, E. H. Bacterial adhesion: modulation by antibiotics which perturb protein synthesis. *Antimicrob. Agents Chemother.* 32:1603–1608, 1988.

Smith, K. E., Besser J. M., Hedberg C. W. *et al.* Quinolone-resistant *Campylobacter jejuni* infections in Minnesota, 1992–1998. *Investigation Team. New Engl. J. Med.* 340:1525–32, 1999.

Spika, J. S., Waterman, S. H., Soo Hoo, G. W. *et al.* Chloramphenicol-resistant *Salmonella newport* traced through hamburger to dairy farms. *N. Engl. J. Med.* 316:565–580, 1987.

Stokstad, E. L. R., and Jukes, T. H. Further observations on the "animal protein factor." *Proc. Soc. Exp. Biol. Med.* 73:523–528, 1950.

Swann, M. M. Joint Committee on the use of antibiotics in Animal Husbandry and Veterinary Medicine. Her Majesty's Stationery Office, London, U.K. 1969.

Chapter 7

Agrios, G. N. *Plant Pathology*, 3rd edition. Academic Press, San Diego, pp. 510–608, 1988.

Aquaculture Outlook, March 14, 2001.

Ervin, M. A. Qualitative use assessment for streptomycin. Document 006306, Environmental Protection Agency, 1988.

Federal Register, August 7, 1996 Docket PF-667: initial filing PP5F4449 vol. 61. No. 153, p. 41154, 1996.

Hirsh, D. C., Ling, G. V., and Ruby, A. L. Incidence of R-plasmids in fecal flora of healthy household dogs. *Antimicrob. Agents Chemother.* 17:313–315, 1980.

Levy, S. B. Antibiotic resistant bacteria in food of man and animals. In: *Antimicrobials and Agriculture* (Woodbine, M., Ed.). Butterworths, London, pp. 525–531, 1983.

McManus, P. S. Antibiotic use in plant disease control. *APUA Newsletter* 1:1–3, 1999.

Monaghan, C., Tierney, U., and Colleran, E. Antibiotic resistance and R-factors in the fecal coliform flora of urban and rural dogs. *Antimicrob. Agents Chemother.* 19:266–270, 1981.

Sheppard, M. E. Antibiotic use in the British Columbia agriculture industry (1996–1998): is the comparison with Norway realistic? *Bull. Agricul. Assoc. Canada* 100:13–16, 1999.

Sundlof, S. F., Riviere, J. E., and Craigmill, A. L. *The Food Animal Residue Avoidance Databank Trade Name File.* Institute of Food and Agricultural Sciences, University of Florida, Gainesville, FL, 1989.

2000 Annual Report on The United States Seafood Industry.

Chapter 8

Baquero, F., Martinez-Beltran, J., and Loza, E. A review of antibiotic resistance patterns of *Streptococcus pneumoniae* in Europe. *J. Antimicrob. Chemother.* 28: Suppl. C:31–38, 1991.

Bush, K. Excitement in the ß-lactamase arena. *J. Antimicrob. Chemother.* 24:831–840, 1989.

Cruciani, R. A., Barker, J. L., Zasloff, M., Chen, H-C., and Colamonici, O. Antibiotic magainins exert cytolytic activity against transformed cell lines through channel formation. *Proc. Natl. Acad. Sci.* (USA) 88:3792–3796, 1991.

Domenico, P., Hopkins, T., and Cunha, B. A. The effect of sodium salicylate on antibiotic susceptibility and synergy in *Klebsiella pneumoniae. J. Antimicrob. Chemother.* 25:343–351, 1990.

Gostin, L. O., Cleary, P. D., Mayer, K. H., Brandt, A. M., and Chittenden, E. H. Screening immigrants and international travelers for the human immunodeficiency virus. *N. Engl. J. Med.* 322:1743–1746, 1990.

Klare, I., Badstubner, D., Konstabel, C. *et al.* Decreased incidence of VanA-type vancomycin-resistant enterococci isolated from poultry meat and from fecal samples of humans in the community after discontinuation of avoparcin usage in animal husbandry. *Microbial Drug Resistance* 5:45–52, 1999.

Kliebe C., Nies, B. A., Meyer, J. F. *et al.* Evolution of plasmid-coded resistance to broad-spectrum cephalosporins. *Antimicrob. Agents Chemother.* 28:302–307, 1985.

Lehrer, R. L., and Ganz, T. Antimicrobial polypeptides of human neutrophils. *Blood* 76:2169–2181, 1990.

Levy, S. B., and Novick, R. P. (Eds.). *Antibiotic Resistance Genes: Ecology, Transfer and Expression.* Cold Spring Harbor, NY, 1986.

Liss, R. H. and Batchelor, F. R. Economic evaluations of antibiotic use and resistance—a perspective report of Task Force 6. *Rev. Infect. Dis.* 9:S297–S312, 1987.

Noble, W. C., Vinary, Z. and Cree, R. G. A. Co-transfer of vancomycin and other resistance genes from *Enterococcus faecalis* NCTC 12201 to *Staphylococcus aureus*. *FEMS Microbiol. Lett.* 93:195–198, 1992.

Skurray, R. A., Rouch, D. A., Lyon, B. R. *et al.* Multiresistant *Staphylococcus aureus:* genetics and evolution of epidemic Australian strains. *J. Antimicrob. Chemother.* 21: Suppl. C: 19–38, 1988.

Tuomanen, E. A single genetic locus on *Bordetella pertussis* controls virulence and tolerance to antibiotics. *APUA Newsletter* 8:4:5, 1990.

Chapter 9

Amidi, S., Solter S., Rashidian, *et al.* Antibiotic use and abuse among physicians in private practice in Shiraz, Iran. *Medical Care* 13:341–345, 1975.

Bosch, X. Household antibiotic storage. *Science* 281:785, 1998.

Chapter 10

Akimitsu, N., Hamamoto, H., Inoue, R. *et al.* Increase in resistance of methicillin-resistant Staphylococcus aureus to beta-lactams caused by mutations conferring resistance to benzalkonium choride, a disinfectant widely used in hospitals. *Antimicrob. Agents Chemother.* 43:3042–43, 1999.

Folberts, G., Walzl, G., Openshaw, P. J. M. Do common childhood infections "teach" the immune system not to be allergic? *Immunol. Today* 21:118–120, 2000.

Levy, S. B. Antibacterial household products: cause for concern. *Emerging Infect. Dis.* 7:S512–515, 2001.

McMurry, L. M., Oethinger, M. and Levy, S. B. Triclosan targets lipid synthesis. *Nature* 394:531–532, 1998.

Schweizer, H. P. Triclosan: A widely used biocide and its link to antibiotics. *FEMS Microb. Lett.* 202:1–7, 2001.

Strachan, D. P. Hay fever, hygiene, and household size. *Brit. Med. J.* 299:1259–60, 1989.

Chapter 11

Annals of Internal Medicine, (antibiotic use in respiratory tract infections) 134:479–529, March 20, 2001.

APUA: Antibiotic resistance: synthesis of recommendations by expert policy groups (1987–2000), 2001.

Farrar, W. E. Jr., and Eidson, M. R factors in strains of *Shigella dysenteriae* type 1 isolated in the Western Hemisphere during 1969–1970. *J. Infect. Dis.* 124:327–329.

Kunin, C. Problems in antibiotic usage. In: *Principles and Practice in Infectious Diseases*, 3rd Edition. (Mandel, G. L., Douglas, R. G. Jr., and Bennett, J. E., Eds.) Churchill Livingstone, New York, pp. 427–434, 1990.

Levy, S. B. Ecology of antibiotic resistance determinants. In: *Antibiotic Resistance Genes: Ecology, Transfer and Expression.* (Levy, S. B., and Novick, R. P., Eds.) Cold Spring Harbor Press, New York, pp. 17–29, 1986.

Levy, S. B. Antibiotic availability and use: consequences to man and his environment. *J. Clin. Epidemiol.* 44:835–875, 1991.

Levy, S. B., Clowes, R. C., and Koenig, E. L. (Eds.). *Molecular Biology, Pathogenicity, and Ecology of Bacterial Plasmids.* Plenum Press, New York, 1981.

Liss, R. H., and Batchelor, F. R. Economic evaluations of antibiotic use and resistance—a perspective report of Task Force 6. *Rev. Infect. Dis.* 9:S297–S312, 1987.

Report of House of Lords Select Committee in Science and Technology (HL Paper 81-I) Resistance to antibiotics and other antibacterial agents. London: The Stationary Office, 1998.

Thamlikitkul, V. Antibiotic dispensing by drug store personnel in Bangkok, Thailand. *J. Antimicrob. Chemother.* 21:125, 1988.

U.K. Standing Medical Advisory Committee, Department of Health, Subgroup on Antimicrobial Resistance. "The path of least resistance." Publications Unit PHLS Headquarters Office, London, 1998.

Walson, J. L, Marshall, B., Pokhrel, B. M. *et al.* Carriage of antibiotic-resistant fecal bacteria in Nepal reflects proximity to Kathmandu. *J. Infect. Dis.* 184:1163–1169, 2001.

WHO Global Strategy for the Containment of Antimicrobial Resistance, 2001.

Index

335

Stuart B. Levy, M.D., is a world renowned authority on antibiotic use and resistance, on which he has written and lectured extensively. He discovered drug efflux as a mechanism for antibiotic resistance and was among the first to document the transfer of drug resistance among animals and people. He is currently Professor of Molecular Biology and Microbiology and of Medicine; Director of the Center for Adaptation Genetics and Drug Resistance at the Tufts University School of Medicine in Boston, Massachusetts; and a staff physician at the New England Medical Center. Dr. Levy is also president of the international *Alliance for the Prudent Use of Antibiotics* and cofounder and Chief Scientific Officer of Paratek Pharmaceuticals, Inc. Profiled in the *New Yorker* for his work on antibiotics, he has also been quoted in all major periodicals and newspapers, including *Time, Newsweek, U.S. News and World Report*, the *New York Times*, the *Washington Post*, and *USA Today*. He has appeared on the *Today Show, Good Morning America, NOVA*, and all major television news networks. Chairperson of a government-sponsored international three-year study of antibiotic use and resistance worldwide, Dr. Levy is the past president of the 42,000-member American Society for Microbiology and received the 1995 Hoechst-Roussel Award for esteemed research in antimicrobial chemotherapy. He was awarded an honorary degree of Doctor in Science from Wesleyan University in 1998 and from Des Moines University in 2001.

Printed in the United States
124108LV00002B/258/P

9 780738 204406